Calories In
Calories Out

Calories In
Calories Out

THE ENERGY-BUDGET WAY TO FITNESS AND WEIGHT CONTROL

by James Leisy

The Stephen Greene Press

Brattleboro, Vermont

Copyright © 1981 by THE STEPHEN GREENE PRESS

This book has been produced in the United States of America. It is designed by IRVING PERKINS ASSOCIATES and published by THE STEPHEN GREENE PRESS, Fessenden Road, Brattleboro, Vermont 05301.

LIBRARY OF CONGRESS CATALOGING IN PUBLICATION DATA

LEISY, JAMES, 1927–
    Calories in/calories out.

    Includes index.
    1. Reducing.   2. Food—Caloric content—Tables.
3. Energy metabolism—Tables.   I. Title.
RM222.2.L4224   613.2   80-22956
ISBN 0-8289-0413-8
ISBN 0-8289-0414-6 (pbk.)

CONTENTS

29/83

FOREWORD

A myocardial infarction at 9:00 A.M. on July 9, 1979, left me with a large amount of leisure and urgent orders to lose 30 pounds. This book is the end result of those converging forces. I was told to count Calories, maintain a negative energy balance and keep a diary. At the bookstores I found Calorie counters that counted only half the Calories, ignoring entirely the minus kind needed to achieve a negative energy balance. Nor were there any diaries available for a fitness and weight control program. By the time I had put together my own diary with both positive and negative Calorie counters I had lost the 30 pounds and acquired a thriving business reprinting diaries for others with the same needs. Fortunately, a representative from the Stephen Greene Press came along to take on the printing and distribution chores, so that you may use this professional copy to get on with your program and I can get back to my leisure.

In addition to acknowledging the contributions of researchers and textbook writers in the fields of medicine, physiology and nutrition, I also wish to express my appreciation to Dr. Sergius Bryner, Dorothy Conway, Alanna Dittoe, Margaret Eastman, Donald Jones, Robert Odell, Paul and Sue Prindle, Dr. Gunnar Sevelius, Jack Thornton, Arthur Weber and Dr. Sheldon Woodward, who read the first draft of this manuscript, offered criticism and suggestions for improvement, and encouraged me in the project. The book is better for their help; any faults that remain are mine alone. Special thanks to Carol Colby, who has always helped to make writing anything an upbeat experience.

PART I

Energy, Fitness and Weight Control

A balanced diet coordinated with regular physical activity is the most effective way to be physically fit and to control your weight. This book integrates information from medical, physiological and nutritional research and focuses it on a systematic fitness and weight control program designed to meet your individual needs and circumstances. It provides a practical, realistic and natural program that allows you to write your own prescription for diet and exercise, eating foods you like and doing activities you enjoy.

Fitness and weight control are functions of the use of energy in your body. If you can control the intake and output of energy, you can control your weight and fitness at desirable levels. Normally this control process should be performed by your body without any conscious effort on your part. But unfortunately, many of today's life-styles tend to frustrate these natural control processes. The solution to this problem is to use your own informed, conscious control to encourage the natural processes to work for you instead of against you.

You will find the information needed for this control in the first part of this book, which is divided into three sections. The first section, entitled "Energy Output," explains the uses of energy by your body and shows how to measure your output of energy and to monitor it from day-to-day on a consistent basis. The second section, entitled "Fitness" (pp. 22–32), explains how to use your output of energy to promote fitness and control your weight. The third section, "Energy Intake" (pp. 32–75), explains how to measure your intake of food and coordinate your diet to achieve your personal goals for weight control.

The second part of the book consists of charts and diary pages which provide a convenient format in which to put this information to work as you learn how your body uses energy, how to count your intake and output of energy, and how to modify your uses of energy to control your weight.

1

YOUR FITNESS AND WEIGHT CONTROL PROGRAM

Specialists in weight reduction recommend that you keep a daily diary summarizing your intake and output of energy. Doing so reinforces your determination to achieve diet goals, of course. But even more importantly, it provides you with a convenient record of what works and doesn't work in your program. The permanent record of your diet and physical activity enables you to re-examine your experiences and re-evaluate your methods (with the help of your medical adviser), make adjustments up or down, as required, and fine-tune your energy control program.

Be sure to undertake this or any weight control program *under the direction and supervision of your medical and nutrition advisers.* Unless your doctor is the one who put this book in your hands, make an appointment to see him or her *now.* Then take this book with you when you keep the appointment, explain your weight loss and fitness objectives, and ask your doctor to help you achieve them.

SECTION I: ENERGY OUTPUT

Your need for energy is second only to the need for air and water. The source of this energy is the food you eat. Most of the food you consume is either burned (oxidized) to meet your current energy requirements or stored for use in the future. If your energy intake is less than you need, your body burns the stored energy and you lose weight. If the intake is more than you need, the excess is stored in your tissues as fat and you gain weight. Under normal living conditions, the stored energy provides a safety margin that can sustain your life for a long period of time without food. Your energy needs are under control when you maintain a proper balance among the three main uses of energy in your body: *energy intake* (food), *energy output* (physical activity and heat) and excess *energy storage* (fat). What is a proper balance? How much excess energy stored as fat is enough? What are appropriate levels for physical activity? What constitutes fitness? Can these factors be measured and rated so that we know where we stand compared to other people or other objective criteria? All of these questions will be answered in the pages that follow.

Measuring Energy Needs

Energy is usually measured in heat units called *calories*. One calorie is the amount of heat required to raise the temperature of one gram of water by one degree Celsius. However, the small calorie used by scientists is too small to be practical for use in measuring energy for our purposes. For this reason, the large kilogram Calorie (abbreviated *kcal.* or *Cal.*), equal to 1000 scientific or small calories, is the preferred measuring unit for food and physical activity,* and is the one used in this book.

The precise amount of energy required varies from individual to individual depending on age, sex, height, weight, physical activity and the influence of these factors on metabolism. The typical range is between 1800 and 3600 Calories daily. It is possible, although not practical, to measure your intake, output and storage of energy on an hour-to-hour basis using various precise measuring devices. Fortunately, it is not necessary to go through this expensive and time-consuming process. You may work out reliably accurate estimates for yourself based on your own particular specifications using the procedures presented in this book.

Body Specifications for Sex, Height and Weight

The first step in determining your daily energy requirement is to specify your ideal maintenance weight. This is the weight you and your doctor agree is best for you. In the final analysis, the choice of an exact ideal or proper weight level is a subjective matter that will be decided and, more importantly, achieved and maintained by you.

According to an old rule of thumb used by doctors, a woman should weigh 100 pounds for her first 5 feet in height plus 5 pounds for each inch over 5 feet. A man should weight 110 pounds for the first 5 feet plus 5 pounds for each inch above. While this rule of thumb is quick and reasonably reliable in many cases, it does not allow for variations in body build, muscular development and other factors that can materially influence

* In 1964, the U.S. National Bureau of Standards adopted the international, or metric system *Joule* as the official energy measurement unit for scientific purposes. If you have a special reason for using the *Joule* instead of the *Calorie*, you may do so by converting numbers according to this formula:

$$1 \text{ Calorie (kcal.)} = 4.184 \text{ kJoules (kJ.)}$$

body weight. A trim, muscular athlete may easily weigh as much or more than a person of the same height who is flabby and out of shape. Therefore, it is desirable to use more precise measurements to determine your ideal weight.

Measuring Body Fat

Most people are overweight because they eat too much and exercise too little. Their energy intake exceeds energy need. The result is an excess of fat stored in the body. Approximately 1 pound of fat is stored for each 3500 Calories of excess energy taken in. We may attack the problem of excess stored fat exclusively through changing our diet. However, this stored fat may also be reduced while maintaining or even gaining weight if the fat is replaced by muscle through a fitness program. Regardless of whether you want to gain, lose or maintain your weight, it is important to know how much body fat you now have. By measuring body fat, instead of body weight, you can arrive at a more precise estimate of your ideal weight.

Ideally, body fat should account for 12 to 15 percent of body weight in men and 22 to 25 percent in women.* Skinfold measurements are the most practical, inexpensive, convenient and, therefore, preferred means of measuring body fat. About half of the fat in the body is located immediately under the skin. Using calipers, or using your finger and thumb as calipers, you can measure the thickness of skinfolds at various locations on your body. These measurements can be used to calculate your excess body fat.

One of the simplest ways to administer and evaluate skinfold measurement was presented by Thomas V. Pipes and Paul A. Vodak of the American College of Sports Medicine.

---

* Body fat may be precisely measured by weighing the body and the water it displaces when immersed. (Body weight in water minus weight of water displaced is proportional to the muscle/fat ratio in the body; lower specific gravity of body indicates a higher proportion of body fat.) You can have this kind of measurement made at a clinic or university fitness center that has the necessary equipment.

Test for Body Composition*

The accuracy of this test in predicting body fat is correlated to your skill and technique in measuring the skinfold. For practice, grasp some skin with your fingers and thumb. Feel around to make sure you are holding only skin and fat and not underlying muscle. The fat will separate easily from the muscle. Once you discover the distinction between the subcutaneous fat and the underlying muscle, lift up a large fold of skin. For proper measurement, press the fold together and measure this thickness to the nearest $\frac{1}{4}$ inch. Practice this technique several times to develop your skill. To improve your accuracy, measure a skinfold and have your husband, wife, children, or friends measure the same skinfold; compare results.

Two separate skinfold sites are necessary to determine your total percentage of body fat. One of the sites differs for men and women. Men and women will both use the right thigh skinfold. Men will also use the abdomen skinfold and women, the skinfold on the back of the upper right arm. We have found that the sites selected relate highest to your overall levels of body fat. The exact locations are described below.

Right thigh skinfold (men and women): While standing, pinch the middle part of the front of the thigh so that the fold is perpendicular to the floor.

Abdomen skinfold (men): While standing, pinch the area just to the right of the navel so that the fold is parallel to the floor.

Right arm (women): Pinch the area behind the middle part of the arm between the shoulder and elbow so that the skinfold is perpendicular to the ground.

1. Measure each skinfold site at least three times. If you are a man, grasp your right thigh and stomach skinfolds firmly. If you are a woman, use your right thigh and arm.

2. From the three measurements calculate the average skinfold for each site and record it on your evaluation score sheet. You will take a total of three measurements for each site and record two measures, or averages.

* From *The Pipes Fitness Test and Prescription.* © 1978 by Thomas V. Pipes and Paul A. Vodak. Reprinted by permission of the publisher, J. P. Tarcher, Inc., 9110 Sunset Boulevard, Los Angeles, California.

Your two skinfold measurements will help you evaluate how much of your body weight is fat. See one of the separate conversion tables for Skinfolds to Body Fat Percentage for men or women, Table 1 or 2. To find your present percentage of body fat, circle the appropriate

TABLE 1 Skinfolds to Body Fat Percentage (Men)

Thigh	¼	½	¾	1	1¼	1½	1¾	2	2¼	2½	2¾	3
3	15	18	20	23	25	27	30	32	35	38	40	43
2¾	14	17	19	22	24	26	29	31	34	37	39	42
2½	13	16	18	21	23	25	28	30	33	36	38	41
2¼	12	15	17	20	22	24	27	29	32	35	37	40
2	11	14	16	19	21	23	26	28	31	34	36	39
1¾	10	.13	15	18	20	22	25	27	30	33	35	38
1½	9	12	14	17	19	21	24	26	29	32	34	37
1¼	8	11	13	16	18	20	23	25	28	31	33	36
1	7	10	12	15	17	19	22	24	27	30	32	35
¾	6	9	11	14	16	18	21	23	26	29	31	34
½	5	8	10	13	15	17	20	20	25	28	30	33
¼	4	7	9	12	14	16	19	21	24	27	29	32

Abdomen

TABLE 2 Skinfolds to Body Fat Percentage (Women)

Thigh	½	¾	1	1¼	1½	1¾	2	2¼	2½	2¾	3
3	33	35	37	39	41	43	45	47	49	51	53
2¾	31	33	35	37	39	41	43	45	47	49	51
2½	29	31	33	35	37	39	41	43	45	47	49
2¼	27	29	31	33	35	37	39	41	43	45	47
2	25	27	29	31	33	35	37	39	41	43	45
1¾	23	25	27	29	31	33	35	37	39	41	43
1½	20	23	25	27	29	31	33	35	37	39	41
1¼	18	20	23	25	27	29	31	33	35	37	39
1	16	18	20	23	25	27	29	31	33	35	37
¾	13	16	18	20	23	25	27	29	31	33	35
½	11	13	16	18	20	23	25	27	29	31	33

Back of Arm

thigh skinfold measurement that appears vertically along the table. Next, look at the values along the bottom of the chart and circle your measurement for the abdomen (men) or the back of the right arm (women). Now draw a horizontal line from your circled thigh skinfold reading and a vertical line from your circled abdomen or arm skinfold reading. The point within the chart at which these two lines intersect is your percentage of body fat.

Evaluation Score Sheet: Body Composition

Right Thigh Skinfold	_____	Inches
Stomach Skinfold (Men)	_____	Inches
Right Arm Skinfold (Women)	_____	Inches
Body Fat Percentage	_____	%

Examine Table 3 to find your fitness zones for body composition. If you carry around more than 18 percent fat (men) or 24 percent fat (women), take a look at Table 4 or 5, ideal weight tables for men and women, pages 8 and 9.

TABLE 3 **Fitness Zones for Body Composition**

Body Fat Percentage

	Danger Zone	*Safety Zone*	*Fitness Zone*
Men	30 29 28 27 26 25	24 23 22 21 20 19 18	17 16 15 14 13 12 11 10
Women	36 35 34 33 32 31	30 29 28 27 26 25 24	23 22 21 20 19 18 17 16

Determining Ideal Body Weight

1. Turn to the Ideal Weight tables for men or women (Table 4 or 5).
2. Circle your present body weight from the numbers to the left of the table.
3. Circle your present percentage of body fat from the numbers along the bottom of the table.
4. Draw a horizontal line from your body weight and a vertical line from your body fat until they intersect.
5. The point at which they intersect is your ideal body weight at 18 percent fat (men) or 24 percent fat (women).

TABLE 4 **Ideal Weight**

(Men at 18% Body Fat)

Present Body Weight

	20	21	22	23	24	25	26	27	28	29	30	31	32	33	34
130	127	125	124	122	120	119	117	116	114	113	111	109	108	106	105
135	132	130	128	127	125	123	122	120	119	117	115	114	112	110	109
140	137	135	133	131	130	128	126	125	123	121	120	118	116	114	113
145	141	140	138	136	134	133	131	129	127	126	124	122	120	118	117
150	146	145	143	141	139	137	135	134	132	130	128	126	124	123	121
155	151	149	147	145	144	143	140	138	136	134	132	130	129	127	125
160	156	154	152	150	148	147	144	142	140	139	137	135	133	131	129
165	161	159	157	155	153	151	149	147	145	143	141	139	137	135	133
170	166	164	162	160	158	155	153	151	149	147	145	143	141	139	137
175	171	169	166	164	162	160	158	156	154	152	149	147	145	143	141
180	176	173	171	169	167	165	162	160	158	156	154	151	149	147	145
185	180	178	176	174	171	169	167	165	162	160	158	156	153	151	149
190	185	183	181	178	176	174	171	169	167	165	162	160	158	155	153
195	190	188	185	183	181	178	176	174	171	169	166	164	162	159	157
200	195	193	190	188	185	183	180	178	176	173	171	168	166	163	161
205	200	198	195	195	190	188	185	183	180	178	175	173	170	168	165
210	205	202	200	197	195	192	190	187	184	182	179	177	174	172	169
215	210	207	205	202	199	197	194	191	189	186	184	181	178	176	173
220	215	212	209	207	204	201	199	196	193	190	188	185	182	180	177
225	220	217	214	211	209	206	203	200	198	195	192	189	187	184	181
230	224	222	219	216	213	210	208	205	202	199	196	194	191	188	185
235	229	226	224	221	218	215	212	209	206	203	201	198	195	192	189
240	234	231	228	225	222	220	217	214	211	208	205	202	199	196	193
245	239	236	233	230	227	224	221	218	215	212	209	206	203	200	197
250	244	241	238	235	232	229	226	223	220	216	213	210	207	204	201
255	249	246	243	239	236	233	230	227	224	221	218	215	211	208	205
260	254	250	247	244	241	238	235	231	228	225	222	219	216	212	209

Present Body Fat Percentage

When you have completed your skinfold measurements and deter-mined your body fat percentage and your ideal maintenance weight, re-cord the results on page 79 in your Fitness and Weight Control Profile. These measurements may be used to establish the goals of your personal-ized weight control program. You may also repeat the measurements pe-riodically to measure the progress of your program.

TABLE 5 **Ideal Weight**

(Women at 24% Body Fat)

	25	26	27	28	29	30	31	32	33	34	35	36	37	38	39
80	79	78	77	76	75	74	73	72	71	69	68	67	66	65	64
85	84	83	82	81	79	78	77	76	75	74	73	72	70	69	68
90	89	88	86	85	84	83	82	81	79	78	77	76	75	73	72
95	94	93	91	90	89	88	86	85	84	83	81	80	79	78	76
100	99	97	96	95	93	92	91	89	88	87	86	84	83	82	80
105	104	102	101	99	98	97	95	94	93	91	90	88	87	86	84
110	109	107	106	104	103	101	100	98	97	96	94	93	91	90	88
115	113	112	110	109	107	106	104	103	101	100	98	97	95	94	92
120	118	117	115	114	112	111	109	107	106	104	103	101	99	98	96
125	123	122	120	118	117	115	113	112	110	109	107	105	104	102	100
130	128	127	125	123	121	120	118	116	115	113	111	109	108	106	104
135	133	131	130	128	126	124	123	121	119	117	115	114	112	110	108
140	138	136	134	133	131	129	127	125	123	122	120	118	116	114	112
145	143	141	139	137	135	134	132	130	128	126	124	122	120	118	116
150	148	146	144	142	140	138	136	134	132	130	128	126	124	122	120
155	153	151	149	147	145	143	141	139	137	135	133	131	128	126	124
160	158	156	154	152	149	147	145	143	141	139	137	135	133	131	128
165	163	161	158	156	154	152	150	148	145	143	141	139	137	135	132
170	168	166	163	161	159	157	154	152	150	148	145	143	141	139	136
175	173	170	168	166	163	161	159	157	154	152	150	147	145	143	140
180	178	175	173	171	168	166	163	161	159	156	154	152	149	147	144
185	183	180	178	175	173	170	168	166	163	161	158	156	153	151	148
190	188	185	183	180	178	175	173	170	168	165	163	160	158	155	153
195	192	190	187	185	182	180	177	174	172	169	167	164	162	159	157
200	197	195	192	189	187	184	182	179	176	174	171	168	166	163	161
205	202	200	197	194	192	189	186	183	181	178	175	173	170	167	165

Present Body Weight

Present Body Fat Percentage

Your Daily Energy Requirement

Having established your ideal body weight, you may now determine how much energy is normally required to maintain your ideal weight on a day-to-day basis. Then, knowing your Daily Energy Requirement, you can use the diary to plan, monitor and control your intake and output of energy in order to reach or maintain your ideal body weight.

The chemical process by which food is converted to energy or potential energy (fat) in your body is called *metabolism*. Your metabolism may be measured and used to establish a reliable guide to your overall Daily Energy Requirements. The energy you burn is used mainly for two purposes:

1. the *internal* work of the body—the vital functions of the heart, lungs, liver, brain, nervous system and so on;
2. the *external* work of your muscles in walking, talking, lifting, pushing or simply in holding up your body to stand or to sit and read.

The *Resting Metabolic Rate* (RMR) measures the energy required to perform the vital internal work of the body that continues at all times, even when you are asleep. This work may account for as much as one-half to three-quarters of your energy needs in a typical day.

Your Resting Metabolic Rate

The estimated Resting Metabolic Rate for your ideal body weight and age is shown in Table 6. When you have located the RMR for your ideal weight and current age in Table 6, circle or check it for convenient reference hereafter, and write it in the space provided in your Fitness and Weight Control Profile, page 79.

Your Physical Activity Rate

You may estimate the remainder of your normal daily energy needs by selecting the occupational group that best describes yours from the following list. Check the appropriate group:

A. *Sedentary:* Sitting most of day; about 2 hours standing or moving about slowly. *Examples:* business executive, airline pilot, songwriter, author, disk jockey.
B. *Light activity:* Sitting or standing much of the day to work with hands; some walking but no strenuous exercise. *Examples:* typist, secretary, teacher, foreman, laboratory worker, taxicab driver, doctor.

TABLE 6 **Resting Metabolic Rate**

Ideal body weight (lbs.)	RMR Ages 21–39	RMR Ages 40–49	RMR Ages 50–59	RMR Ages 60–69	RMR Age 70 and over
75	816	792	767	734	694
80	864	838	812	778	734
85	936	908	880	842	796
90	984	954	925	886	836
95	1032	1001	970	929	877
100	1080	1048	1015	972	918
105	1152	1117	1083	1036	979
110	1200	1164	1128	1080	1020
115	1248	1211	1173	1123	1061
120	1296	1257	1218	1166	1102
125	1368	1327	1286	1231	1163
130	1416	1374	1331	1274	1204
135	1464	1420	1376	1318	1244
140	1536	1490	1444	1382	1306
145	1584	1536	1489	1426	1346
150	1632	1583	1534	1469	1387
155	1680	1630	1579	1512	1428
160	1752	1699	1647	1577	1489
165	1800	1746	1692	1620	1530
170	1848	1793	1737	1632	1571
175	1896	1839	1782	1706	1612
180	1968	1909	1850	1771	1673
185	2016	1956	1895	1814	1714
190	2064	2002	1940	1858	1754
195	2136	2072	2008	1922	1816
200	2184	2118	2053	1966	1856
205	2232	2165	2098	2009	1897
210	2280	2212	2143	2052	1938
215	2352	2281	2211	2117	1999
220	2400	2328	2256	2160	2040
225	2448	2375	2301	2203	2081
230	2496	2421	2346	2246	2122
235	2568	2491	2414	2311	2183
240	2616	2538	2459	2354	2224
245	2664	2584	2504	2398	2264
250	2736	2654	2572	2462	2326
255	2784	2700	2617	2506	2366
260	2832	2747	2662	2549	2407
265	2880	2794	2707	2592	2448
270	2952	2863	2775	2657	2509
275	3000	2910	2820	2700	2550

    C. *Moderate activity:* Mostly walking and standing while working; very little sitting. *Examples:* housewife and mother, actress, gardener, light industry worker, carpenter, farmer, salesman.

    D. *Strenuous activity:* Vigorous and extended physical activity much of the working day; little sitting. *Examples:* professional dancer, skater, unskilled laborer, forester.

    E. *Very strenuous activity:* Extended, vigorous and very competitive sports or physical work; little sitting. *Examples:* professional tennis, swimming, basketball, football, lumbering.

Now compute your estimated *Daily Energy Requirement* by inserting your RMR in the appropriate blank for the group you have chosen and by completing the multiplication as indicated. Use the rate most appropriate to your typical level of vigor (low, moderate, high, very high).

Group
                    Level of Vigor

A. Multiply: _____ × $\begin{matrix} 1.2 \\ 1.3 \\ 1.4 \\ 1.5 \end{matrix}$ = _____
         (Your RMR)   (Daily Energy Requirement)

B. Multiply: _____ × $\begin{matrix} 1.3 \\ 1.4 \\ 1.5 \\ 1.6 \end{matrix}$ = _____
         (Your RMR)   (Daily Energy Requirement)

C. Multiply: _____ × $\begin{matrix} 1.4 \\ 1.5 \\ 1.6 \\ 1.7 \end{matrix}$ = _____
         (Your RMR)   (Daily Energy Requirement)

D. Multiply: _____ × $\begin{matrix} 1.7 \\ 1.8 \\ 1.9 \\ 2.0 \end{matrix}$ = _____
         (Your RMR)   (Daily Energy Requirement)

E. Multiply: _____ × 2.0 = _____
         (Your RMR)   (Daily Energy Requirement)

If you belong to Group D or E, your doctor may advise an upward adjustment in the formula, particularly if you are underweight. In Group A, B or C, a downward adjustment may be needed, especially if you are overweight. No matter which group you belong to, your doctor may suggest adjustments to fit your particular circumstances. Variations in individual requirements within groups can be broad, depending on the vigor with which a person works, the amount of time devoted to the activities involved and special circumstances in one's health and habits.

When you have confirmed your estimated Daily Energy Requirement with your doctor, write it in the appropriate space in your Energy Output Summary on page 82. While this figure does not give you a precise measurement of your actual daily energy needs, it does give you a "working" estimate that should be reasonably close to the actual and, more importantly, *one that may be verified or adjusted by keeping records and studying results in your diary.*

Suppose, for example, that you are a 50-year-old, 5'11" business executive with an ideal weight of 167 pounds and a Resting Metabolic Rate of 1692 Calories. You might elect to use the lowest level of vigor to describe your typical daily output and, therefore, calculate an estimated Daily Energy Requirement of 2030 Calories.

$$\frac{1692}{\text{(Your RMR)}} \times \frac{1.2}{\text{(lowest level)}} = \frac{2030}{\text{(Daily Energy Requirement)}}$$

On the other hand, if you chose the highest level of vigor to describe your daily output, you would estimate 2538 Calories to be your Daily Energy Requirement.

$$\frac{1692}{\text{(Your RMR)}} \times \frac{1.5}{\text{(highest level)}} = \frac{2538}{\text{(Daily Energy Requirement)}}$$

The 508 Calorie difference between these two estimates could make a significant difference in your weight control program, as much as a pound gained or lost each week (7 days × 500 Calories per day = 3500 Calories or 1 pound per week).

To avoid this costly kind of error and to understand better the uses of energy in your body, you should: (1) begin keeping a daily log of your actual energy output in physical activity (see Diary, Day 1, page 94); and (2) learn to use the Energy Output Table (pages 15–19).

Preparing and Using the Energy Output Table

To count the Calories you expend in daily physical activities, the Energy Output Table (pages 15–19) must be personalized. To complete it:

1. Read through the activities listed in the first column and check (✔) each one that is identical or similar to one which you do.
2. Check (✔) the corresponding *Resting Metabolic Rate* (RMR) in the second column that is closest to your RMR. This number will be the same for each activity listed throughout the table.
3. Check (✔) the number in the third column which corresponds to the RMR checked. This number will vary for each activity listed throughout the table.

The number of Calories per hour checked for each activity represents your own personal energy cost for each hour invested in the activity listed or one similar to it. The Energy Output Table was derived from specific, controlled research studies collated by J.V.G.A. Durnin and R. Passmore.* Additional activities are listed in the Physical Activities Index that follows the table (see page 20). You may wish to add some of these activities to the table by writing them in at the levels suggested. Also, you may wish to make some common-sense adjustments to adapt the data to your personal level of energy use. For example, driving an automobile with automatic gear shift in commuter traffic daily for an hour or two might easily be a regular event for you. This activity is probably more similar to "piloting an aircraft" at activity level 1.4 than it is to driving occupationally with a manual shift at activity level 2.3. Using the latter Calories per hour count would probably substantially overstate your energy output cost on a daily basis. If this is true for you, you should add "driving automobile" at level 1.4 of your Energy Output Table.

In using the Energy Output Table it is important to think of it only as a guide. It is difficult to estimate *output* with the same degree of accuracy as *food intake* values. Nevertheless, you can, with time and practice, and by profiting from the errors you make with estimates, learn to count energy output fairly accurately.

---

* J.V.G.A. Durnin and R. Passmore, *Energy, Work, and Leisure* (London: Heinemann Educational Books, 1967); and R. Passmore and J.V.G.A. Durnin, "Human Energy Expenditure," *Physiol. Rev.* 35:801 (1955).

TABLE 7

ENERGY OUTPUT TABLE

Level	Activity	RMR (Daily)	Calories per Hour (Rounded)	Level	Activity	RMR (Daily)	Calories per Hour (Rounded)
1.0	Resting					1584	92
	Sleeping or	1152	48			1656	97
	lying at ease.	1224	51			1728	101
		1296	54			1800	105
		1368	57			1872	109
		1440	60			1944	113
		1512	63			2016	118
		1584	66				
		1656	69	1.7			
		1728	72		Sitting,	1152	82
		1800	75		typing with electric	1224	87
		1872	78		typewriter,	1296	92
		1944	81		using desk calculator.	1368	97
		2016	84		Standing and moving	1440	102
1.2	Very Light Work				around an office.	1512	107
	Sitting at ease while	1152	58		Playing cards.	1584	112
	listening to music,	1224	61		Playing woodwind	1656	117
	reading,	1296	65		instruments.	1728	122
	hand sewing,	1368	68			1800	128
	knitting.	1440	72			1872	133
		1512	76			1944	138
		1584	79			2016	143
		1656	83	1.9			
		1728	86		Lower range of domestic	1152	91
		1800	90		and light industrial work;	1224	97
		1872	94		e.g., cleaning shoes,	1296	103
		1944	97		paring vegetables,	1368	108
		2016	101		cooking,	1440	114
1.4	Very Light Work				painting indoors,	1512	120
	Sitting and writing,	1152	67		typing using mechanical	1584	125
	doing office desk work.	1224	71		typewriter.	1656	131
	Repairing watches.	1296	76			1728	137
	Piloting an aircraft.	1368	80			1800	143
	Milking by machine.	1440	84			1872	148
		1512	88			1944	154
						2016	160

15

ENERGY OUTPUT TABLE, Continued

Level	Activity	RMR (Daily)	Calories per Hour (Rounded)	Level	Activity	RMR (Daily)	Calories per Hour (Rounded)
2.1					bakery tasks,	1440	150
	Sitting and eating.	1152	101		canoeing 2.5 mph.	1512	158
	General laboratory work.	1224	107		Horseback riding at a walk.	1584	165
		1296	113			1656	173
		1368	120			1728	180
		1440	126			1800	188
		1512	132			1872	195
		1584	139			1944	203
		1656	145			2016	210
		1728	151				
		1800	158				
		1872	164	**2.7**			
		1944	170		Walking 2 mph on the	1152	130
		2016	176		level.	1224	138
					Dusting, setting a dinner	1296	146
2.3	**Light Work**				table, washing dishes by	1368	154
	Lower range of work in	1152	110		hand.	1440	162
	transportation, building	1224	117		Hanging wallpaper.	1512	170
	trades, mechanized agri-	1296	124			1584	178
	culture and forestry; e.g.,	1368	131			1656	186
	driving a car or truck	1440	138			1728	194
	with manual shift, or a	1512	129			1800	203
	combine harvester;	1584	152			1872	211
	planting by machine,	1656	159			1944	219
	sharpening a saw.	1728	166			2016	227
	Playing piano or stringed	1800	173				
	instrument.	1872	179				
	Playing billiards.	1944	186	**2.9**			
		2016	193		Walking 2 mph on the	1152	139
					level, with a 22-pound	1224	148
2.5					load.	1296	157
	Upper range of light	1152	120		Walking 2.5 mph on the	1368	165
	industrial work;	1224	128		level.	1440	174
	e.g., assembly work,	1296	135		Personal care; e.g., dressing,	1512	183
	machine sewing,	1368	143		bathing.	1584	191

Level	Activity	RMR (Daily)	Calories per Hour (Rounded)
	Lowest range of agricultural work; e.g., troweling, transplanting.	1656	200
		1728	209
		1800	218
	Repairing shoes.	1872	226
	Operating a lathe.	1944	235
	Playing a pipe organ.	2016	244
3.1	Milking by hand.	1152	149
	Weeding and raking.	1224	158
	Playing volleyball.	1296	167
		1368	177
		1440	186
		1512	195
		1584	205
		1656	214
		1728	223
		1800	233
		1872	242
		1944	251
		2016	260
3.5 Moderate Work	Walking 3.1 mph on the level.	1152	168
		1224	179
	Light janitorial work, industrial laundry, garage mechanics.	1296	189
		1368	200
		1440	210
	Washing a car.	1512	221
	Bowling.	1584	231
		1656	242
		1728	252
		1800	263
		1872	273
		1944	284
		2016	294

Level	Activity	RMR (Daily)	Calories per Hour (Rounded)
3.7	Walking 3.1 mph on the level, with a 22-pound load.	1152	178
		1224	189
		1296	200
	Bed-making, vacuuming, scrubbing (kneeling).	1368	211
		1440	222
	Cutting wood with power saw.	1512	233
		1584	244
		1656	255
		1728	266
		1800	278
		1872	289
		1944	300
		2016	311
4.0	Hoeing and weeding.	1152	192
	Window-cleaning.	1224	204
	Cycling at 5.5 mph.	1296	216
	Playing with children.	1368	228
	Table tennis.	1440	240
		1512	252
		1584	264
		1656	276
		1728	288
		1800	300
		1872	312
		1944	324
		2016	336
4.5	Cutting hedge by hand.	1152	216
	Outdoor painting, plastering.	1224	230
		1296	243
	Swimming leisurely, golf, archery.	1368	257
		1440	270

ENERGY OUTPUT TABLE, Continued

Level	Activity	RMR (Daily)	Calories per Hour (Rounded)
		1512	284
		1584	297
		1656	311
		1728	324
		1800	338
		1872	351
		1944	365
		2016	378
5.0			
	Walking 2 mph up a 10% grade.	1152	240
	Dancing a waltz.	1224	255
		1296	270
		1368	285
		1440	300
		1512	315
		1584	330
		1656	345
		1728	360
		1800	375
		1872	390
		1944	405
		2016	420
6.0			
	Climbing stairs.	1152	288
	Shoveling (18-pound load	1224	306
	thrown 3.28 ft. ten times	1296	324
	per minute).	1368	342
	Canoeing 4 mph,	1440	360
	tennis,	1512	378
	skiing downhill and using	1584	396
	towbar uphill,	1656	414
	cycling 10 mph.	1728	432
		1800	450
		1872	468

Level	Activity	RMR (Daily)	Calories per Hour (Rounded)
		1944	486
		2016	504
6.5			
	Walking 2 mph up a 20% grade.	1152	312
	Cutting hardwood with hand saw.	1224	332
		1296	351
		1368	371
		1440	390
		1512	410
		1584	429
		1656	449
		1728	468
		1800	488
		1872	507
		1944	527
		2016	546
7.0 Heavy Work			
	Digging pit in soil.	1152	336
	Felling, trimming and	1224	357
	barking trees.	1296	378
	Weight lifting.	1368	399
	Swimming leisurely under	1440	420
	water, wearing fins and	1512	441
	wet suit.	1584	462
		1656	483
		1728	504
		1800	525
		1872	546
		1944	567
		2016	588
7.5			
	Upper range of manual	1152	360

Level	Activity	RMR (Daily)	Calories per Hour (Rounded)
	work in agriculture and	1224	383
	in building, mining and	1296	405
	steel industries.	1368	428
	Hockey, basketball, football	1440	450
	(game average).	1512	473
		1584	495
		1656	518
		1728	540
		1800	563
		1872	585
		1944	608
		2016	630
8.0			
	Chopping with axe with	1152	390
	1.28 kg. head, 35 blows	1224	408
	per minute.	1296	432
	Skiing on level over hard	1368	456
	snow, 3.7 mph.	1440	480
	Horseback riding at a	1512	504
	gallop.	1584	528
	Dancing actively, country	1656	552
	or folk style.	1728	576
		1800	600
		1872	624
		1944	648
		2016	672
9.0			
	Cross-country running.	1152	432
	Climbing, light load and	1224	459
	slope.	1296	486
	Swimming strenuously.	1368	513
	Boxing.	1440	540
		1512	567
		1584	594

Level	Activity	RMR (Daily)	Calories per Hour (Rounded)
		1656	621
		1728	648
		1800	675
		1872	702
		1944	729
		2016	756
10.0			
	Climbing, heavy load and	1152	480
	slope.	1224	510
	Heaviest occupational work.	1296	540
	Football and squash during	1368	570
	play.	1440	600
		1512	630
		1584	660
		1656	690
		1728	720
		1800	750
		1872	780
		1944	810
		2016	840
15.0			
	Walking in loose snow with	1152	720
	a heavy pack.	1224	765
	Skiing uphill at maximum	1296	810
	speed.	1368	855
	Swimming strenuously	1440	900
	under water with full	1512	945
	gear.	1584	990
	Bicycle racing.	1656	1035
		1728	1080
		1800	1125
		1872	1170
		1944	1215
		2016	1260

Physical Activities Index to Energy Output Table

This index presents in alphabetical order the activities listed by energy output level in the Energy Output Table. The numbers after each item indicate, from low to high, the levels of energy output at which each activity is rated. The numbers in parentheses indicate activities not listed in the Table because controlled research studies were not available when the Table was originally compiled. The levels in parentheses are believed to be comparable to the ratings of the earlier studies.

Agricultural trades, 2.3, 2.9, 4.0, 4.5, 6.0, 7.5
Archery, 4.5
Assembly work, 2.5
Auto repair, 3.5

Badminton (3.1)
Baseball (1.7, 5.0)
Basketball, 7.5
Bathing, 2.9
Bed-making, 3.7
Benchwork, standing (2.5)
Bicycling, 4.0, 6.0, 15.0
Billiards, 2.3
Boating, 1.4
Bowling, 3.5
Boxing, 9.0
Brick laying (3.7)
Building trades occupations, 2.3, 4.5, 7.5

Calisthenics:
   abdominal exercises (4.5, 5.0)
   arm-swinging, hopping (4.5, 5.0, 8.0)
   balancing (4.5, 5.0)
   trunk bending (4.5, 5.0)
Canoeing, 2.5, 6.0
Car washing, 2.3
Carpentry, 2.3
Chopping with axe, 8.0
Climbing, 6.0, 9.0, 10.0
Cooking, 1.9
Croquet (1.7)
Cross-country running, 9.0
Cutting hedge, wood, 3.7, 6.5
Cycling, 4.0, 6.0, 15.0

Dancing, 5.0, 8.0
Desk work, 1.4
Digging, 6.0, 7.0
Domestic work, 1.9, 2.7, 3.7
Dressing, 2.9
Driving, 1.4, 2.3
Dusting, 2.7

Eating, 2.1
Exercise (see Calisthenics)

Factory assembly work, 2.5
Farm work, 2.3, 2.9, 4.0, 4.5, 6.0, 7.5
Felling trees, 7.0
Fencing (5.0, 8.0)
Flying, 1.4
Football, 7.5, 10.0
Forestry, 2.3, 7.0

Garage mechanics, 3.5
Gardening, 2.3, 2.9, 3.1, 4.0, 4.5, 6.0
Golf, 4.5
Gymnastics (see Calisthenics)

Handball (6.0, 10.0)
Hand sewing, 1.2
Hanging wallpaper, 2.7
Heavy industrial work, 10.0
Hiking, 2.0, 2.7, 2.9, 3.5, 3.7, 5.0, 6.5, 15.0
Hockey, 7.5
Hoeing, 4.0
Horseback riding, 2.5
Housework, 1.2, 1.4, 1.9, 2.3, 2.7, 2.9, 3.1, 3.5, 3.7, 4.0

Ice hockey, 7.5
Ice-skating, 7.5
Indoor games, sitting, 1.7
Ironing (2.3)

Janitorial work, 3.5
Jogging (2.7 to 8.0)
Judo (9.0, 10.0)

Karate (9.0, 10.0)
Kitchen activity, standing and moving, 1.9
Kneeling to work, 3.7
Knitting, 1.2

Laboratory work, 2.1
Laundry work, industrial, 3.5
Light industrial work, 1.9, 2.5
Listening, sitting, 1.2
Lying at ease, 1.0

Mechanics, 3.5
Milking, 1.4, 3.1
Mining, 7.5
Mopping floors (3.7)
Motorcycling (2.5)

Office work, sitting, 1.4
Office work, standing and moving, 1.7
Operating machinery, 1.4, 1.7, 2.9, 3.7

Painting, 1.9, 4.5
Personal care; e.g., dressing, bathing, 2.9
Piano playing, 2.3
Piloting aircraft, 1.4
Ping pong, 4.0
Pipe organ playing, 2.9
Planting, 2.3
Plastering, 4.5
Playing games, 1.7, 4.0
Playing musical instruments, 1.7, 2.3, 2.9
Preparing food, 1.9

Raking, 3.1
Racquetball, 6.0
Reading, 1.2
Repair work, 1.4, 2.9
Roller skating (6.0)

Rope jumping (8.0)
Rowing:
  51 strokes per min. (4.0)
  87 strokes per min. (6.0)
  97 strokes per min. (9.0)
Running, 9.0

Scrubbing, kneeling, 3.7
Setting a dinner table, 2.7
Sewing, domestic, 1.2
Sewing, industrial, 2.5
Sharpening a saw, 2.3
Shoe repair, 2.9
Sitting, 1.2
Shoveling, 6.0
Skating (6.0)
Skiing, 6.0, 8.0, 15.0
Sleeping, 1.0
Soccer (7.5)
Softball (5.0)
Squash, 10.0
Standing and moving around, 1.7
Steel industry trades, 7.5
Stringed instrument playing, 2.3
Swimming, 4.5, 7.0, 9.0, 15.0

Table tennis, 4.0
Telephoning, 1.2
Tennis, 6.0
  doubles (5.0)
Transportation industry trades (e.g., driving), 2.3
Trimming trees, 7.0
Typing, 1.7, 1.9

Vacuuming, 3.7
Volleyball, 3.1

Walking, 2.7, 2.9, 3.5, 3.7, 5.0, 6.5, 15.0
Wallpaper hanging, 2.7
Washing a car, 3.5
Watching TV or movie (1.2)
Weeding, 3.1, 4.0
Weight lifting, 7.0
Window cleaning, 4.0
Wrestling (9.0)
Writing, sitting, 1.5

SECTION II: FITNESS

You can maintain a negative energy balance and control your weight by limiting the intake of energy in your diet (as discussed in the next section), by increasing the output of energy through physical activity (as discussed in this section), or by a combination of both approaches. The advantage of including a fitness program in your life-style is that it allows you to eat more than you would otherwise be able to enjoy. This approach is especially appealing if you have a hearty appetite and enjoy any kind of physical activity. By simply inserting a 30-minute walk into your daily energy exchange, you may lose from 5 to 10 pounds in a year's time and improve your health in the process, without spending one cent on special clothing or equipment.

Physical fitness can be quantified and its benefits can be measured and predicted. Most important of all, it is available to *everyone, not just athletes.* You do not have to compete with anybody to achieve fitness. You may accomplish it privately, if you wish.

Exercise physiologists stress three basic guidelines for measuring the fitness effects of exercise: *frequency, duration* and *intensity.* Regarding frequency and duration, there seems to be widespread agreement that fitness training requires that you exercise regularly a minimum of three times weekly for periods of at least 20 to 30 minutes. There is less agreement about intensity. Some exhort us to put forth maximum effort, while others plead for lower levels of effort with more frequent and longer exercise periods. When the main objectives are conditioning and weight control however, and especially for those who are substantially overweight and out of condition, it is generally agreed that exercise should begin at lower levels of intensity and work up to higher levels slowly and methodically.

Your doctor can help you determine the extent of physical activity that is both safe and desirable for you. An exercise stress test, in which you pedal a stationary bicycle or walk a treadmill at various degrees of difficulty while your heart and blood pressure are monitored, can provide information on your present condition that may be used to design your fitness program and conduct it safely. In addition to alerting you to any special medical problems, your doctor can use the stress test to verify your maximal attainable heart rate and your recommended target zone for fitness activity. This is the zone of intensity or vigor in physical activity which conditions the muscles and cardiovascular system without being overly strenuous.

Recommended Zones for Pulse-Rated Exercise

The maximal attainable heart rate for most people is directly related to age, and may be estimated by subtracting your age in years from 220. Table 8 (below and p. 24) shows maximal attainable heart rates and target zone ranges for pulse-rated exercise for normal, active adults. (Note how these rates decrease steadily with age.) Exercise physiologists recommend more frequent and longer workouts at lower pulse rates (between 50 and 60 percent of maximum intensity) for fat weight reduction programs. For cardiovascular fitness programs your doctor may also recommend workouts at pulse rates between 50 and 60 percent. Some recommend even higher rates (up to the 70 to 85 percent level), though many physicians believe these upper ranges should be used only by athletes while in training.

TABLE 8 **Pulse-Rated Exercise**

Age	Maximum Heart Rate	50% of Maximum Rate	60% of Maximum Rate	70% of Maximum Rate	75% of Maximum Rate	80% of Maximum Rate	85% of Maximum Rate
21	199	100	119	139	149	159	169
22	198	99	119	139	149	158	168
23	197	99	118	138	148	158	167
24	196	98	118	137	147	157	167
25	195	98	117	137	146	156	166
26	194	97	116	136	146	155	165
27	193	97	116	135	145	154	164
28	192	96	115	134	144	154	163
29	191	96	115	134	143	153	162
30	190	95	114	133	143	152	161
31	189	95	113	132	142	151	161
32	188	94	113	132	141	150	160
33	187	94	112	131	140	150	159
34	186	93	112	130	140	149	158
35	185	93	111	130	139	148	157
36	184	92	110	129	138	147	156
37	183	92	110	128	137	146	156

TABLE 8, **Continued**

Age	Maximum Heart Rate	50% of Maximum Rate	60% of Maximum Rate	70% of Maximum Rate	75% of Maximum Rate	80% of Maximum Rate	85% of Maximum Rate
38	182	91	109	127	137	146	155
39	181	91	109	127	136	145	154
40	180	90	108	126	135	144	153
41	179	90	107	125	134	143	152
42	178	89	107	125	134	142	151
43	177	89	106	124	133	142	150
44	176	88	106	123	132	141	150
45	175	88	105	123	131	140	149
46	174	87	104	122	131	139	148
47	173	87	104	121	130	138	147
48	172	86	103	120	129	138	146
49	171	86	103	120	128	137	145
50	170	85	102	119	128	136	145
51	169	85	101	118	127	135	144
52	168	84	101	118	126	134	143
53	167	84	100	117	125	134	142
54	166	83	100	116	125	133	141
55	165	83	99	116	124	132	140
56	164	82	98	115	123	131	139
57	163	82	98	114	122	130	139
58	162	81	97	113	122	130	138
59	161	81	97	113	121	129	137
60	160	80	96	112	120	128	136
61	159	80	95	111	119	127	135
62	158	79	95	111	119	126	134
63	157	79	94	110	118	126	133
64	156	78	94	109	117	125	133
65	155	78	93	109	116	124	132
66	154	77	92	108	116	123	131
67	153	77	92	107	115	122	130
68	152	76	91	106	114	122	129
69	151	76	91	106	113	121	128
70	150	75	90	105	113	120	128
71	149	75	89	104	112	119	127
72	148	74	89	104	111	118	126
73	147	74	88	103	110	118	125
74	146	73	88	102	110	117	124
75	145	73	87	102	109	116	123

In the final analysis, you should choose the pulse-rate target zone that enables you to condition your muscles and cardiovascular system with a vigor and intensity appropriate to your physical condition but one that is safe and not overly strenuous. By concentrating on physical activity in your target zone you can get the best result for the least effort. When you have verified your maximal attainable heart rate and target zone for fitness activity with your doctor, write these numbers in the designated spaces of your personal Fitness and Weight Control Profile on page 79.

The next and obvious questions are: When and where to begin? Once you have been cleared by your doctor, there is no reason to wait any longer. And the nicest thing about fitness training is that you can do it wherever you are and whenever you wish. For calisthenics your bedroom or hotel room will do nicely when you get up in the morning or before you go to bed at night. To walk, open a door and go. These when and where questions are easily answered. But we should take a little more time to decide *what* to do and *why*. Goals are important in fitness activity because you should design the program to get the results you want.

Establishing Fitness Goals

Most people wish to be generally fit for health, social recreation and sports (dancing, boating, tennis, stand-up parties and so on), as well as for the requirements of their occupations and for weight control. We shall confine our recommendations to these goals and suggest sources of additional information for those who wish to pursue other specific training objectives.

Planning Your Fitness Program

You can achieve a high degree of cardiovascular fitness (as much as an 80 percent improvement over your present condition) with a surprisingly small investment of effort in as short a period as 30 days. The main thing is to get started. Don't wait for the "right" day. Start today.

Any exertion beyond minimum effort is a step in the right direction. Any use of the muscles stimulates development. If you are sitting while you read this, stand. If you are standing, move around. When you use an automobile, park it farther from your destination, instead of closer, and walk briskly the rest of the way. Climb stairs in preference to riding elevators. Stand up for telephone conversations instead of sitting. *Constantly seek opportunities to upgrade the level and load of all your physical activities.* This is the simplest and fastest way to get a fitness program going without making any basic change in your life-style. As you begin to discover these fitness opportunities, you may want to keep a special Fitness Log in the spaces provided in your diary.

Measuring Progress

A Fitness Log is a good place to keep measurement records (your weight, pulse, pinch test results, etc.) so that you can monitor your progress toward goals and objectives. You are more likely to reach your goals when you keep a daily record and make adjustments in your program as needed.

It is not at all necessary or even desirable to begin a fitness program with great effort and intensity. In fact, that is a good way to nip your program in the bud. Progressive loading of effort and difficulty is the age-old, proven method of fitness training, whether for Olympic athletes or middle-aged retreads. Start out with as much time as you can spare easily and at a comfortable pace and work your way up from there. For openers, you might simply start walking for 5, 10 or 15 minutes a day at 2 mph, and then start "loading" the speed and/or distance and/or time allotted per week, working your way up to walking say 3 or 4 miles in an hour daily.

The serious fitness training begins when you start putting in enough physical effort to get your pulse rate into your target zone and keep it there for a sustained period of time. At least 20 to 30 minutes of sustained effort at any dynamic physical activity (see page 31) that keeps your pulse rate up in your target zone will normally have a significant effect on your cardiovascular system and promote fitness. The upper limit to the intensity of your activity should not be surpassed and certainly need not be sustained. The time spent in the target zone should be sandwiched between warm-up and cool-down periods of 5 to 10 minutes, during which you engage in the same physical activity but at a much slower and less intense pace. These warm-ups and cool-downs are essential to prepare your joints and muscles for both the beginning and ending of the activity so that you will avoid soreness, injuries and blood circulation problems. You will, of course, need to learn how to read your pulse accurately in order to accomplish these results and record the results in your diary.

How to Count Your Pulse Rate

There are several locations at which you may count your pulse conveniently and which you may learn to find with reasonable ease by yourself, or with a little help from your doctor or nurse, if needed. These locations include:

1. The radial artery on the thumb side of your wrist near the base of your thumb joint.
2. The carotid artery on either side of your throat, just below your jaw or above your collarbone and in front of the vertical strip of muscle on the side of the neck.
3. The temporal artery at the side of your head just in front of your ear.

One location is about as good as another for counting your pulse at rest. However, most people seem to prefer the wrist for quick fitness counts, especially considering the juggling of the watch that is involved. Here is how to take the wrist pulse:

1. Turn your wristwatch so that you can see the face when looking at the palm of your hand.
2. Wrap your other hand around the wristwatch hand so that the tips of the fingers rest on the pulsating artery between the palm of the hand and the face of the watch (see the illustration on the next page).
3. When you feel the pulse under your finger start counting the beats, with zero, as your second-hand crosses a marker.
4. When your second-hand reaches a 6-second marker, stop and multiply by 10 to get your pulse rate per minute. Or you may

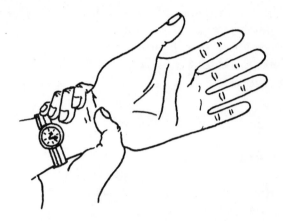

prefer to take the count at 10 seconds on your watch and multiply by 6 to get the pulse rate per minute. Both methods are used.

At rest you may let the second-hand sweep to a full minute as you count, and check your count against the intermediate points at 6 and 10 seconds on the watch. In this way you can compare and test the accuracy of your shorter counts.

The short fitness count, which sacrifices a degree of accuracy, is necessary when you interrupt a physical activity to make a quick measurement before your pulse rate decreases. The fall-off rate after exercise is too great to provide an accurate reading at 1 minute, or even at the 15-second point used by most doctors and nurses for a resting pulse.

Counting your pulse is a little awkward at first, but becomes quite easy to do with continued practice. Once you are able to take your pulse with confidence you may wish to record your pulse rate in your daily Fitness Log for specific times before, during and after your fitness workouts. For example, you might stop for pulse counts at these times:

1. While resting prior to exercise warm-up.
2. While standing without moving around prior to warm-up.
3. At the end of the 5- to 10-minute warm-up.
4. At 5-minute intervals during the intensive period of effort in order to keep within your target zone.
5. At the end of the 5- to 10-minute cool-down.
6. While resting after your workout.

Your objectives for these pulse ratings might include one or both of the following:

1. *Lowering of your normal resting pulse rate.* Fitness lowers the resting pulse rate, and should do so observably within a period of 30 days after your conditioning program begins. Lowering by 5 to 10 points is not unusual. Resting pulse rates per minute normally average between 72 and 76 beats for men, and between 75 and 80 beats for women. However, since both higher and lower rates can be normal, you should discuss any deviations from the norm with your doctor. Generally speaking, a lower resting pulse rate is healthier and better for your heart muscle and decreases the risk of coronary disease.

2. *Gradually increasing exercise tolerance until the pulse rate reaches and stays within your target zone during the 20- to 30-minute period of more intensive effort.* Any movement is better than none. However, in most instances you should reach a minimum pulse rate of 50 percent of your maximum heart rate during the intense portion of your exercise to improve cardiovascular fitness. Levels of improvement may be raised at 30- or 60-day intervals up to a maximum rate allowed by your doctor.

As stated earlier, exercise tolerance is increased by the process known as loading or overloading, which may be accomplished in various ways. The three most common methods of loading are to *increase:*

1. *Intensity.* Lift a heavier load, move faster or move against heavier resistance.
2. *Duration.* Hold the load longer or move farther.
3. *Frequency.* Do the same thing, but do it more often.

To use walking as an example, your program might be loaded this way:

First period (30 days): Walk 15 minutes at 2 mph once daily.
Second period (30 days): Walk 15 minutes at 2 mph twice daily.
Third period (30 days): Walk 30 minutes at 2 mph twice daily.
Fourth period (30 days): Walk 30 minutes at 2.5 mph twice daily.
Fifth period (30 days): Walk 30 minutes at 3 mph twice daily.

Thereafter you might continue to increase the load every 30 days by walking faster, then switching to jogging at 4 mph, and then eventually to running. Or, additional loading could be accomplished by adding a backpack with increasing amounts of sand in it. Also you could start walking up grades at increasing rates. When you have exhausted the loading possibilities of one form of exercise you can switch to another. Some people prefer more variety anyhow. For example, walking on Monday, Wednesday and Friday; riding a bicycle on Tuesday, Thursday and Saturday; golf on Sunday.

Others prefer to exercise alone in their own room. In *Total Fitness in 30 Minutes a Week*, Laurence E. Morehouse (the exercise physiologist from the University of California at Los Angeles who worked with the problems of astronauts in space) prescribes a set of "cabin exercises" that can be done anywhere, including your bedroom or hotel room.° These easy exercises, used in graded sets of difficulty, begin with *pushaways* from the wall to build the muscles of your shoulders, chest and arms, *sitbacks* (sit-ups in reverse) to expand the muscles of the abdomen and back, and 5 minutes of pulse-rated *fitness hops* "danced" while you whistle a tune or turn on the radio. The objective of these daily exercise sets is to build muscle mass, endurance and strength (in that order). They may also be used privately to prepare your body for more public and sporty activities. The author also includes conditioning exercises for specific sports: tennis, bowling, swimming, golf, softball and skiing.

Not all forms of exercise are equally good for fitness training. What counts toward fitness is the way in which the exercise challenges the cardiovascular system. The best fitness exercises are rhythmic, continuous, sustained workouts in which the muscles pump repetitively, tensing and then relaxing. These cardiovascular fitness exercises are called *isotonic* or *dynamic* in contrast to *isometric* exercises, like weight lifting, in which muscles are shortened, bunched, tensed. Isotonic exercise promotes the flow of blood instead of inhibiting it. Isometric exercise has its purposes for building athletic strength and skill, but it does not promote stamina or endurance or build cardiovascular fitness to the same degree. Your fitness exercise should also be *aerobic*. An aerobic exercise is one that steadily feeds oxygen to the muscles for the duration of the exercise period. These are the exercises that can be sustained for longer periods of time and do

° Laurence E. Morehouse and Leonard Gross. *Total Fitness in 30 Minutes a Week* (New York: Pocket Books, 1975).

not leave you huffing and puffing and exhausted at completion.

Here is the list of activities which, properly done, may be used effectively for graded, pulse-rated personal programs to develop cardiovascular fitness:

Walking°	Climbing
Jogging°	Running°
Dancing	Rope jumping or skipping
Rowing	Skating
Isotonic calisthenics	Skiing
Isotonic gymnastics	Swimming
Cycling	

Skill sports and games like golf, tennis, handball and squash may be played vigorously and with some fitness benefit. However, they have many limitations: The play is stop and go in nature. The acquisition of skill offsets effort instead of promoting it. Social play may be too relaxed, while competitive play can be dangerous to people with cardiac problems. There is a potential for accidents and injuries that can be detrimental to fitness. The emphasis can be on isometric instead of isotonic exercise. And, finally, measurements of fitness results (e.g., pulse rate) are awkward to accomplish during such activities. Nevertheless, if you prefer these sports and are healthy, do them. You will be more likely to continue an activity you enjoy. After your game, add an aerobic session. Such activity will increase your stamina and benefit your skill sport.

There are excellent books that present graded fitness programs involving various activities and sports which may be used effectively with your diary. Among them are:

COOPER, KENNETH M., and BROWN, KEVIN. *Aerobics.* New York: M. Evans and Company, 1968. (Also available in a paperback edition from Bantam Books.)

COOPER, KENNETH M. *The Aerobics Way.* New York: M. Evans and Company, 1977. (Also available in a paperback edition from Bantam Books.)

PIPES, THOMAS V., and VODAK, PAUL A. *The Pipes Fitness Test and Prescription.* Los Angeles: J. P. Tarcher, Inc., 1978.

° Walking, jogging and running qualify as independent dynamic activities. They may also be considered together as phases in a continuum of increasing intensity (e.g., walking up to 4 mph, jogging up to 6 mph, running over 6 mph).

Regularity and longevity are important. To be effective, your program should be conducted at least three times weekly with no more than two days elapsing between workouts. Whether you conduct your program alone or with a group is strictly a matter of personal preference. Either way works. Results begin to show in a week or two, and by 4 to 6 weeks measurable improvement in fitness will be felt. Your body will become more efficient, you will sleep better and you will have a feeling of greater vitality and strength. Assuming you continue to upgrade your program and vary it to use both arms and legs, you will achieve all-round fitness in 3 to 6 months. Thereafter, fitness can be maintained by regular workouts at the level you have reached. If you cut back the level or frequency of your workouts, you will begin to decondition. As much as half of your fitness can be lost in a few weeks. If your program is interrupted by illness or unavoidable circumstances, you should resume the program at a lower level and gradually work your way back to where you were.

Biofeedback is the name we have given to the process by which your body signals whether things are going well or badly. We have discussed some of the positive signals: better sleep, vitality and strength. If your body sends negative signals, you should stop or slow down and discuss the signals with your doctor. Here is a list of warning signals (in descending order of concern):

Abnormal, irregular, rapid or slow pulse rate.

Pain, ache or pressure in chest, arm, shoulder, throat or jaw.

Dizziness, lightheadedness, inability to coordinate.

Nausea or vomiting.

Prolonged recovery (e.g., rapid heartbeat or breathlessness continues 5 to 10 minutes after exercise stops).

Muscle, bone or joint fatigue (e.g., cramps, shin splints, charley horse, gout, arthritis).

Prolonged fatigue and/or insomnia.

SECTION III: ENERGY INTAKE

Fitness contributes to your health, but it cannot do the whole job by itself. What you eat also has much to do with the state of your health. Since whatever you eat *is* your diet, it is important to have some understanding of how diet relates to fitness and health as well as to weight control.

Diets and Dieting Goals

Just as your physical activity can be designed and coordinated for fitness objectives, your diet can also be organized to accomplish particular objectives. In addition to weight control goals, your diet should be designed to provide a healthy, balanced supply of the nutrients needed for body functions and activities, including oxidation for energy, building or maintenance of body tissues and the regulation of body processes. The nutrient ratio in Calories should consist of 12 to 15 percent protein, no more than 35 percent fat and the rest carbohydrates.° Saturated fats and sucrose (table sugar) should be avoided. Fortunately, a wide variety of foods promotes better nutrition.

The prevention or care of diabetes and cardiovascular, renal, gastrointestinal and various other diseases and specific health problems should be important considerations in establishing diet objectives. You may also wish to consider specific athletic objectives in formulating your diet. Pregnancy has unique dietary concerns. In addition to these and other special matters that vary from person to person, most of us like to eat foods we enjoy in company with people we like in normal situations. That is, we do not want to be force fed, isolated or ostracized because of a special diet. After considering all of these factors, and any others pertinent to your situation, and discussing them with your doctor and dietician, you should write down your dietary goals and note any special requirements on page 79 in your Fitness and Weight Control Profile.

Recommendations for Low-Calorie Diets

Any diet regimen may be used with your diary program. A convenient comparative analysis of diet prescriptions is available in *Rating the Diets* by Theodore Berland and the editors of *Consumer Guide®* (New York:

° Dieticians generally agree on these ratios and principles of nutrition, though there is some variation among recommendations. The American Heart Association has recommended a diet of 15% protein, 34% fat and 51% carbohydrates. A widely followed diet program developed by E. S. Gordon and others at the University of Wisconsin Medical School is high in protein (30%; 400 Calories), moderate in fat (55%; 720 Calories) and low in carbohydrates (15%; 200 Calories).

New American Library, 1979). Though each formula or prescription diet may emphasize some distinctive or "miracle" feature, the basic pattern is usually centered around low-Calorie selections of essential foods and nutrients that add up to between 1000 and 1500 Calories a day. You may, of course, find a planned diet that happens to fit you well individually, but most of these mass-market diets have the disadvantage of impersonal menu selection, dishes requiring unusual or inconvenient preparation, monotonous and limited food selection, isolation of the dieter from friends and family and the real world, and a general lack of freedom, flexibility and individual interest.

Many physicians and nutritionists recommend that motivated dieters construct their own reducing diets within guidelines that provide good nutrition while restricting the intake of energy at lower levels. This approach has the advantages of permitting a personal choice of menus and real-world flexibility in addition to providing an opportunity to learn good food habits that can last a lifetime. If you decide to construct your own diet, you will find the summary of diets and dietary considerations shown in Table 9 useful.

TABLE 9 **Basic Low-Calorie Diet Summary**

Food Categories	Recommended Servings Daily	Calories Per Serving		Low Cal. Diet	
		Low	High	Low	High
1. Breads, cereals	3	50	75	150	225
2. Dairy: milk, cheese, eggs	2	80	100	160	200
3. Polyunsaturated fats	3	50	75	150	225
4. Fruit	2	50	100	100	200
5. Meat, fish, game	2 (3 oz. each)	150	300	300	600
6. Vegetables (including soups, salads)	7+	20	50	140	350
Total intake of Calories				1000	1800
Typical output of Calories				−2000	−2800
Daily energy balance				−1000	−1000

This table summarizes the recommendations of most dieticians for balanced, nutritious, low-Calorie diets on which dieters can maintain a negative daily energy balance of up to −1000 Calories and lose up to 2 pounds of fat weight a week. By following these recommendations consistently you should receive the nutrients—but not the Calories—you need to meet the Recommended Daily Dietary Allowances of the United States, Canada and most countries throughout the world. According to these standards, the typical moderately active male has an energy output of 2800 Calories daily and the female 2000. Using Table 9 you may adjust your energy intake up or down to meet your own diet goal based on your own specific Daily Energy Requirement. These adjustments may be made by reducing or increasing the size of the servings allowed. (The number of servings should not be changed without consulting your doctor.) Your doctor can also advise you as to the need for iron and other supplementary vitamins and minerals which may be required at the lowest energy intake levels or for long-term diets.

The recommended servings and food categories shown in the table represent a balanced, varied supply of dairy products, meat, fruit, cereals and vegetables. The first two columns indicate nutritionists' recommendations for daily servings in each food category. The next two columns indicate the number of Calories recommended per serving for low-Calorie diets, ranging from a low of 1000 Calories to a high of 1800 Calories per day. The *Energy Intake Table* (pages 38 through 67) in this book lists a broad variety of foods that meet these specifications.

Measuring Daily Energy Intake

To keep your food intake in balance with your energy output you simply log the food you eat and count the Calories consumed, then adjust either your intake or output to balance. To maintain your present weight, if it is the desired weight, you plan food intake that equals your estimated Daily Energy Requirement, as adjusted from time to time to reflect your actual daily energy output. If you wish to lose weight, you may plan your meals more carefully to reduce your intake until you have reached your desired weight.

To lose fat without increasing physical activity, you must reduce intake by at least 3500 Calories for each pound of fat you wish to lose. If you reduce your intake by 500 Calories a day, you may lose fat at the rate of 1 pound per week, at least initially, and at the rate of 3 pounds or more a month over a longer period of time (because weight reduction lowers metabolism). If you reduce intake by 1000 Calories per day, you may lose 2 pounds of fat a week initially, and 6 pounds a month or more over a longer period. In addition to reducing fat weight, you will usually experience a certain amount of weight loss due to a decrease in body fluids, especially in the beginning stages of a weight loss diet. While this easy and dramatic weight loss can be encouraging to the novice dieter (the phenomenon supports a large industry of quick-result fad diet purveyors), it is advisable to concentrate on the more lasting long-term results which are earned slowly but surely through a day-by-day attrition of excess body fat.

EXAMPLE 1

Energy Input Log	Cal.
Break: ☐ Orange Juice 4	80
Bran Flakes - 1 cup	105
Non-fat Milk - 8 oz	90
Coffee - black	0
Lunch: ☐ Tuna Sandwich	300
Salad (Lettuce -10; 1 T. Fe. Dr. 75)	85
(Cott. Ch., 1/3 cup -80; Tom. 40)	120
Pill Pickle	15
Iced Tea	—
Dinner: ☐ Consomme	20
Waldorf Salad	150
Chicken, 1/2 Broiler	240
Veg. Spinach -25 Beets -30, Gr. Beans -20	75
Fresh Pear, Coffee Black	100
Fitness Log	

		Total In (+)	1380
		Total Out (−)	2395
		Balance (±)	−1015

☑ = check when medication is taken.

To log your food intake, simply list the name and quantity of each food you eat throughout the day in the Energy Intake Log of your diary. Then look up the energy value in Calories of each food item in the Energy Intake Table (pages 38–67) and write this in on your log after each food item. At the end of the day add up the total to determine your energy intake for the day. Then subtract the Energy Output total for the day to arrive at your Energy Exchange Balance for the day. A plus balance means you are gaining weight, a minus balance means you are losing.

Example 1 shows a typical Energy Intake Log.

Energy Intake Table

You should now be ready to carry out your personalized fitness and weight control program, using the diary pages at the back of this book. The Energy Intake Table that follows should provide an invaluable resource for you. This table was designed specifically for use with this fitness and weight control program. It is based on chemical analyses of foods and calculated values compiled for the U.S. Department of Agriculture under the direction of Bernice K. Watt and Annabel L. Merrill, supplemented by various independent food studies. The data shown are representative values. Careful consideration was given to variations in food products due to variety, breed, stage of maturity, seasonal and geographic differences and production, storage, trimming, manufacturing, preparation and handling practices. We believe this table presents more accurate, comparative and systematically useful and detailed information in a more convenient format than has customarily been made available. All Caloric values in the table are rounded both systematically and comparatively for ease in counting and effectiveness in results. All counts are based on edible portions ready-to-serve, unless otherwise stated in the table.

Following the Intake Table are tables of the weights and measures commonly used with foods, and a section on tips and suggestions for dieters. You may wish to glance through this information before going on to complete the summaries for your program that appear in Part II of this book.

TABLE 10

ENERGY INTAKE TABLE

	Typical Measure	Calories (Rounded)		Typical Measure	Calories (Rounded)
Appetizers and Snacks°			Pate de foie gras	1 T.	60
Anchovies, pickled	5 fillets	35	Peanut butter	1 T.	95
Anchovy paste	1 t.	15	Popcorn:		
Carrots, raw, sliced	½ cup	25	Plain	1 cup	25
Caviar, granular	1 T.	42	Sugar-coated	1 cup	135
Caviar, granular	1 oz.	74	With oil and salt	1 cup	40
Caviar, pressed	1 T.	54	Potato chips	each	10
Caviar, pressed	1 oz.	90	Pretzels:	per oz.	110
Celery, raw, 4 average			Logs		
stalks or 1 cup, chopped	4 oz.	20	(3″ long, ½″ diam.)	10	195
Cheese spread, American,			Rods		
pasteurized	1 T.	40	(7½″ long, ½″ diam.)	each	55
Clam dip, sour cream	1 t.	10	Sticks		
Clams, 4 cherrystones or			(3⅛″ long, ⅛″ diam.)	10	25
5 littlenecks	2½ oz.	55	Twists, Dutch		
Corn chips (e.g., Fritos)	per oz.	165	(2¾ × 2⅝ × ⅝″)	each	65
Franks, smoked	each		Twists, one-ring		
(1¾″ long, ⅝″ diam.)	(⅓ oz.)	30	(1½″ diam.)	10	80
Ham, deviled	1 T.	45	Twists, thin		
Ham, baked or smoked	per oz.	105	(3¼ × 2¼ × ¼″)	10	235
Ham, canned	per oz.	55	Twists, three-ring		
Herring, pickled	per oz.	65	(1⅞ × 1¾ × ¼″)	10	120
Liver paste	1 T.	60	Shrimp:		
Lobster paste	1 t.	15	Large (10 shrimp:		
Olives, small (see Salads			3¼″ long)	2 oz.	70
for detailed listing)	each	5	Medium (10 shrimp:		
Onion dip, sour cream	1 T.	30	2½″ long)	1(+) oz.	40
Oysters, Atlantic°°	each	15	Small (10 shrimp:		
Oysters, Pacific, small°°	each	25	2″ long)	⅗ oz.	20
Oysters, Pacific, large°°	each	45	Shrimp paste	1 t.	15
			Snails, meat only	per oz.	25
			Tuna:		
			Packed in oil,		
			drained solids (2 T.)	per oz.	55
			Packed in water (2 T.)	per oz.	35

° See also separate listings for breads, crackers, dairy products, fruit, meat, fish and game, nuts and dried seeds, etc.
°° Tomato sauce = 20 Cal.

	Typical Measure	Calories (Rounded)		Typical Measure	Calories (Rounded)
Tuna, cont.:			Whiskeys (Bourbon,		
Raw (2 T.)	per oz.	40	blended, Canadian, gin,		
Salad (2 T.)	per oz.	50	Irish, rum, rye, Scotch,		
Turkey, light meat			tequila, vodka, etc.):		
without skin			80 proof	per oz.	65
$(4 \times 2 \times \frac{1}{4}'')$	1½ oz.	75	86 proof	per oz.	70
			90 proof	per oz.	75
			94 proof	per oz.	80
Beverages, Alcoholic°			100 proof	per oz.	85
Distilled Liquors:			**Malt Liquors:**°°		
Brandy	per oz.	75	Ale	12 oz.	150
Cognac	per oz.	75	Beer, regular	12 oz.	150
Liqueurs:			Beer, light	12 oz.	100
Anisette	per oz.	110	Stout	12 oz.	120
B & B	per oz.	95	**Mixed drinks:**°°°		
Benedictine	per oz.	115	Bloody Mary	6 oz.	120
Cherry Heering	per oz.	80	Daiquiri	3 oz.	130
Creme d' almonde	per oz.	100	Eggnog	4 oz.	365
Creme de banane	per oz.	95	Gimlet	4 oz.	125
Creme de cacao	per oz.	100	Gin and tonic	8 oz.	190
Creme de cassis	per oz.	85	Hot toddy	8 oz.	165
Creme de menthe	per oz.	110	Irish coffee	8 oz.	265
Curacao	per oz.	100	Mai tai	8 oz.	275
Drambuie	per oz.	110	Manhattan, dry	3 oz.	140
Kirsch	per oz.	85	Manhattan, sweet	3 oz.	160
Kummel	per oz.	75	Margarita	3 oz.	140
Maraschino	per oz.	95	Martini, traditional		
Peppermint Schnapps	per oz.	85	3-to-1	3 oz.	130
Pernod	per oz.	80	Martini, dry	3 oz.	135
Rock & Rye	per oz.	95	Martini, extra dry	3 oz.	140
Sloe gin	per oz.	85	Milk punch	10 oz.	285
Southern Comfort	per oz.	120			
Tia Maria	per oz.	95			
Triple Sec	per oz.	85			

° Actual measures may vary from pony (1 oz.) to jigger (1½ oz.)

°° Malt liquors: Actual measures vary from 8 oz. glass to 12 oz. can or bottle to pint or 16 oz. stein.

°°° Mixed drinks: Typical measures and Calories based on standard ingredients.

ENERGY INTAKE TABLE, Continued

	Typical Measure	Calories (Rounded)		Typical Measure	Calories (Rounded)
Beverages, Alcoholic, Cont. *			Wines, cont.:		
			Dubonnet	4 oz.	160
Mint julep	12 oz.	210	Madeira	4 oz.	190
Moscow mule	8 oz.	145	Malaga	4 oz.	175
New Orleans gin fizz	8 oz.	170	Marsala	4 oz.	160
Old fashioned cocktail	4 oz.	180	Moselle	4 oz.	80
Piña colada	6 oz.	185	Muscatel	4 oz.	180
Planter's punch	16 oz.	225	Port	4 oz.	180
Pousse cafe	3 oz.	75	Retsina	4 oz.	80
Ramos fizz	8 oz.	170	Rhine	4 oz.	95
Rusty nail	4 oz.	215	Rhone	4 oz.	95
Salty dog	8 oz.	180	Riesling	4 oz.	90
Sangria	10 oz.	210	Rosé	4 oz.	100
Screwdriver	6 oz.	175	Sauterne	4 oz.	100
Side car	3 oz.	115	Sherry, dry	4 oz.	165
Silver fizz	8 oz.	170	Sherry, cream	4 oz.	200
Stinger	3 oz.	150	Sylvaner	4 oz.	90
Tom and Jerry	8 oz.	345	Table wine, dry	4 oz.	100
Tom Collins	12 oz.	160	Table wine, sweet	4 oz.	155
Whiskey highball	8 oz.	175	Tokay	4 oz.	100
Whiskey sour	6 oz.	145	Vermouth, French	4 oz.	120
Zombie	14 oz.	350	Vermouth, Italian	4 oz.	190
Wines:			Zinfandel	4 oz.	100
Apple	4 oz.	155			
Barbera	4 oz.	100	**Beverages, Non-Alcoholic**		
Beaujolais	4 oz.	95	Acerola juice	6 oz.	45
Bordeaux	4 oz.	95	Apple juice	6 oz.	80
Burgundy, red	4 oz.	95	Apricot nectar	6 oz.	100
Burgundy, sparkling	4 oz.	115	Blackberry juice	6 oz.	65
Burgundy, white	4 oz.	90	Blueberry juice	6 oz.	95
Cabernet	4 oz.	100	Carrot juice	6 oz.	35
Chablis	4 oz.	90	Cider	6 oz.	80
Champagne	4 oz.	100	Clam juice	8 oz.	50
Chardonnay	4 oz.	90	Club soda	8 oz.	0
Chenin blanc	4 oz.	90	Cocoa (with milk)	8 oz.	200
Chianti	4 oz.	100	Coffee, ** hot or iced	8 oz.	0
Claret	4 oz.	95			

* Actual measures may vary from pony (1 oz.) to jigger (1½ oz.)

** Sugar: 1 t. = 15 Cal.; 1 t., rounded = 25 Cal. Milk: 1 oz. = 40 Cal. Cream: 1 oz. = 65 Cal. Non-dairy cream substitute: 1 T. = 35 Cal.

	Typical Measure	*Calories (Rounded)*		*Typical Measure*	*Calories (Rounded)*
Colas	8 oz.	90	Tomato juice	6 oz.	35
Cranberry juice	6 oz.	110	Tonic water	8 oz.	70
Cream sodas	8 oz.	100	Vegetable juice	6 oz.	30
Fig juice	6 oz.	80			
Fruit-flavored ades			**Breads**••		
(e.g., lemonade)	8 oz.	100			
Fruit-flavored sodas			Bagel, two halves		
(e.g., orange crush)	8 oz.	105	(3½″ diam.)	1 oz.	150
Ginger ale	8 oz.	70	Banana bread	2 oz.	150
Ginger beer	8 oz.	70	Biscuit		
Grape juice	6 oz.	120	(2″ diam., ¼″ high)	1 oz.	100
Grapefruit juice	6 oz.	70	Blueberry muffin		
Hot chocolate	8 oz.	200	(2⅜″ diam., 1½″ high)	1⅖ oz.	110
Lemon juice	per oz.	7	Boston brown bread		
Lemon juice	6 oz.	40	(3″ diam., ½″ high)	1¼ oz.	75
Lime juice	per oz.	8	Bran raisin bread		
Lime juice	6 oz.	45	(1 slice: ¾″ thick)	1⅔ oz.	150
Loganberry juice	6 oz.	90	Bran muffin		
Milk drinks (*see*			(2⅝″ diam., 1⅜″ high)	1⅖ oz.	105
Dairy Products)			Breadcrumbs, dry,		
Mineral waters	8 oz.	0	grated (1 cup)	3½ oz.	395
Nectarine juice	6 oz.	110	Bread sticks		
Orange juice	6 oz.	80	(4 to 7″ long)	⅙ oz.	40
Ovaltine	8 oz.	150	Bread sticks, Vienna		
Papaya juice	6 oz.	65	(6½″ long, 1¼″ wide)	1¼ oz.	105
Passion fruit juice	6 oz.	155	Cinnamon bun,		
Pear nectar	6 oz.	90	with raisins	2 oz.	165
Pineapple juice	6 oz.	95	Coffee cake		
Postum, hot or iced°	8 oz.	15	(4½″ diam.)	3 oz.	250
Quinine water	8 oz.	70	Cloverleaf roll		
Raspberry juice, red	6 oz.	60	(2½″ diam., 2″ high)	1 oz.	85
Root beer	8 oz.	95	Danish pastry:		
Sauerkraut juice	6 oz.	15	Large, plain (4¼″ diam.,		
Tangerine juice	6 oz.	75	1″ high)	2¼ oz.	275
Tea, hot or iced°	8 oz.	0	With fruit or nuts	2½ oz.	350
			Small, plain (3⅛″)	1½ oz.	180
			With fruit or nuts	1¾ oz.	225

° Sugar: 1 t. = 15 Cal.; 1 t., rounded = 25 Cal.
Milk: 1 oz. = 40 Cal. Cream: 1 oz. = 65 Cal.
Non-dairy cream substitute: 1 T. = 35 Cal.
Lemon juice: 1 oz. = 7 Cal.

•• Butter or margarine: 1 t. = 35 Cal.; Jams, jellies, preserves: 1 t. = 20 Cal.

ENERGY INTAKE TABLE, Continued

	Typical Measure	*Calories (Rounded)*
Breads, Cont.°		
Date nut bread	2 oz.	150
Dinner rolls:		
Cloverleaf roll (2½″ diam., 2″ high)	1 oz.	85
Hard roll, round (3¾″ diam., 2″ high)	1¾ oz.	155
Hard roll, rectangular (3¾ × 2½ × 1¾″)	1 oz.	80
Parkerhouse (2⅜ × 2 × 1⅜″)	1 oz.	75
Doughnut, cake, large (3⅝″ diam., 1¼″ high)	2 oz.	225
Doughnut, cake, small (1½″ diam., ¾″ high)	½ oz.	55
Doughnut, yeast-leavened (3¾″ diam., 1¼″ high)	1¼ oz.	175
English muffin (3½″ diam.)	1 oz.	150
Flat bread (wafer: 2 × 4½″)	5 wafers	100
French bread (5 × 2½ × 1″)	1¼ oz.	100
Small (2½ × 2 × ½″)	½ oz.	45
Gingerbread (2¾ × 2¾ × 1⅜″)	2 oz.	175
Hamburger bun (3½″ diam.)	1½ oz.	120
Hot dog bun (6″ long, 2″ wide, 1½″ high)	1½ oz.	120
Italian bread (large slice: 4½ × 3¼ × ¾″)	1 oz.	85
Italian bread (small slice: 3¼ × 2½ × ½″)	⅓ oz.	30
Melba toast (½ slice: 3½ × 2″)	⅒ oz.	15
Pancake (4″ diam.)	1⅗ oz.	100
Popover	1¾ oz.	115
Pumpernickel (regular slice: 5 × 4 × ⅜″)	1(+) oz.	80
Pumpernickel (snack slice: 2½ × 2 × ¼″)	¼ oz.	20
Raisin bread (3¾ × 3⅝ × ½″)	1 oz.	65
Roman meal bread (3¾ × 3⅝ × ½″)	1 oz.	75
Rye bread (regular slice: 4¾ × 3¾ × ½″)	1 oz.	60
Rye bread (snack slice: 2½ × 2 × ¼″)	¼ oz.	25
Soya bread (3¾ × 3⅝ × ½″)	1 oz.	65
Sweet roll (4¼″ diam., 1″ high)	2¼ oz.	275
Tortilla (6″ diam.)	1 oz.	65
Vienna bread (4¾ × 4 × ½″)	1 oz.	75
Waffle (7″ diam.)	2½ oz.	210
White bread (regular slice: 4⅜ × 4 × ½″)	1 oz.	75
White bread (sandwich slice: 4 × 4 × ½″)	¾ oz.	65
Whole wheat (4 × 4 × ½″)	1 oz.	60
Zwieback	¼ oz.	35
Breakfast Cereals		
All-Bran	1 cup	190
Alpha-Bits	1 cup	110
Apple Jacks	1 cup	110
Bran	1 cup	145
Wheat germ added	1 cup	180

° Butter or margarine: 1 t. = 35 Cal.; Jams, jellies, preserves: 1 t. = 20 Cal.

	Typical Measure	Calories (Rounded)		Typical Measure	Calories (Rounded)
Bran flakes, 40% bran	1 cup	105	Rice, granulated, cooked	1 cup	125
Bran flakes with raisins	1 cup	145	Rice Honeys	1 cup	150
Cap'n Crunch	1 cup	150	Rice Krispies	1 cup	105
Cheerios	1 cup	110	Rice, puffed	1 cup	60
Cocoa Krispies	1 cup	115	Honey or cocoa added	1 cup	140
Cocoa Puffs	1 cup	110	Rice, shredded	1 cup	100
Corn flakes	1 cup	100	Special K	1 cup	70
Corn flakes, sugar-coated	1 cup	155	Stars	1 cup	110
Corn grits, cooked	1 cup	125	Sugar Frosted Flakes	1 cup	145
Corn, puffed	1 cup	80	Sugar Pops	1 cup	110
Corn, puffed,			Sugar Smacks	1 cup	110
sweetened	1 cup	115	Total	1 cup	110
Cocoa flavored	1 cup	120	Trix	1 cup	110
Fruit flavored	1 cup	120	Wheat and malted		
Corn, shredded	1 cup	100	barley, cooked	1 cup	160
Cream of Wheat	1 cup	130	Instant cooking,		
Farina, instant cooking,			cooked	1 cup	200
cooked	1 cup	155	Wheat flakes	1 cup	105
Farina, regular or quick			Wheat germ	1 T.	25
cooking, cooked	1 cup	105	Wheat, puffed	1 cup	55
Fruit Loops	1 cup	115	With sugar or sugar		
Grape Nut Flakes	1 cup	150	and honey added	1 cup	135
Grape Nuts	1 cup	440	Wheat, rolled, cooked	1 cup	180
Jets	1 cup	140	Wheat, shredded:		
Kix	1 cup	85	Biscuit (3¾ × 2¼ × 1″)	each	90
Life	1 cup	140	Biscuits, spoon-size		
Lucky Charms	1 cup	100	(1 × ⅝ × ⅜″)	1 cup	175
Oat flakes	1 cup	165	Bite-size squares	1 cup	200
Oat granules, maple-			Round biscuit		
flavored, cooked	1 cup	150	(3″ diam. × 1″)	each	70
Oatmeal or rolled oats,			Shreds	1 cup	145
cooked	1 cup	135	Wheat, whole-meal,		
Oats, puffed	1 cup	100	cooked	1 cup	110
Oats with corn, puffed	1 cup	140			
Oats, shredded	1 cup	170	**Condiments and Relishes°**		
OK's	1 cup	80	Capers	1 T.	5
Pep	1 cup	105	Chicory leaves	10	5
Post Toasties	1 cup	110	° *See also* Salads and Salad Ingredients, Sauces		
Product 19	1 cup	105	and Gravies.		

ENERGY INTAKE TABLE, Continued

	Typical Measure	Calories (Rounded)		Typical Measure	Calories (Rounded)
Condiments and Relishes, Cont. *			Barbecue-flavored		
			($1\frac{7}{8} \times \frac{3}{16}$")	$\frac{1}{10}$ oz.	15
Chili sauce, tomato	1 T.	15	Butter ($1\frac{7}{8} \times \frac{3}{16}$")	$\frac{1}{10}$ oz.	15
Chives, chopped	1 T.	1	Butter, rectangular		
Chutney	1 T.	50	($2\frac{1}{2} \times 1\frac{3}{8} \times \frac{1}{8}$")	$\frac{1}{7}$ oz.	20
Citron	1 oz.	90	Cheese-flavored		
Coconut, dried, shredded	1 T.	40	($1\frac{7}{8} \times \frac{3}{16}$"):	$\frac{1}{10}$ oz.	15
Garlic clove			Rectangular sticks		
($1\frac{1}{4} \times \frac{5}{8} \times \frac{3}{8}$")	1 clove	5	(10 crackers: $1\frac{5}{8} \times \frac{1}{4}$")	$\frac{1}{3}$ oz.	45
Ginger root, candied	1 oz.	95	Round		
Ginger root, fresh	1 oz.	13	($1\frac{7}{8}$" diam., $\frac{3}{16}$" thick)	$\frac{1}{8}$ oz.	20
Grapefruit peel, candied	1 oz.	90	Square (10 crackers:		
Herbs and spices	dash	0	$1 \times \frac{1}{8}$" thick)	$\frac{2}{5}$ oz.	50
Horseradish	1 T.	5	Corn chips (e.g., Fritos)	1 oz.	165
Mustard	1 t.	5	Graham:		
Parsley, raw sprig			Chocolate coated		
($2\frac{1}{2}$") or chopped	2 T.	5	($2\frac{1}{2} \times 2 \times \frac{1}{4}$")	$\frac{1}{2}$ oz.	65
Peanut butter	1 T.	95	Plain (2 squares: $2\frac{1}{2}$")	$\frac{1}{2}$ oz.	55
Pepper, black	1 t.	5	Crumbed	1 cup	
Pepper, hot, chili	2 t.	15		(3 oz.)	325
Pickle relish	1 T.	20	Sugar–honey		
Pimientos	per oz.	8	($5 \times 2\frac{1}{2} \times \frac{3}{16}$")	$\frac{1}{2}$ oz.	60
Salt	sprinkle	0	Crumbed	1 cup	
Vinegar	1 T.	2		(3 oz.)	350
Water chestnuts (5 to					
7 corms: $1\frac{1}{2}$" diam.)	4 oz.	70	Matzoh	$\frac{1}{10}$ oz.	15
Watercress, chopped	$\frac{1}{2}$ cup	12	Oyster	per oz.	115
Watercress sprigs with			Rusk ($3 \times \frac{1}{2}$")	$\frac{1}{4}$ oz.	40
stems	7 sprigs	5	Rye (2×3")	$\frac{1}{7}$ oz.	25
			Saltines (2" sq.)	$\frac{2}{5}$ oz.	50
			Sandwich, cheese or		
Crackers and Chips			peanut butter (4)	1 oz.	140
			Soda:		
Animal, 10 crackers	1 oz.	115	Biscuit (2" sq.)	$\frac{2}{5}$ oz.	15
Arrowroot ($1\frac{7}{8} \times \frac{3}{16}$")	$\frac{1}{10}$ oz.	15	Crumbed	1 cup	
Bacon-flavored				($2\frac{1}{2}$ oz.)	310
($1\frac{7}{8} \times \frac{3}{16}$")	$\frac{1}{10}$ oz.	15	Soup or oyster (10)	$\frac{1}{3}$ oz.	35
			Whole-wheat (2" sq.)	$\frac{2}{5}$ oz.	25
* *See also* Salads and Salad Ingredients, Sauces and Gravies.			Zweiback	per oz.	120

	Typical Measure	Calories (Rounded)		Typical Measure	Calories (Rounded)
Dairy Products			Cheese, cont.:		
			Liederkranz	1 oz.	85
Butter or margarine	1 pat		Limburger	1 oz.	100
(1¼″ square)	(⅕ oz.)	35	Monterey Jack	1 oz.	105
Butter or margarine	1 t.		Mozzarella	1 oz.	85
	(⅕ oz.)	35	Muenster	1 oz.	100
Butter or margarine	1 T.		Parmesan	1 oz.	110
	(½ oz.)	100	Grated	1 T.	23
			Pimiento		
Cheese:			(3½ × 3⅜ × ⅛″)	1 oz.	105
American			Ricotta	1 oz.	45
(2¾ × 2¼ × ¼″)	1 oz.	100	Romano	1 oz.	110
Blue (2¾ × 2½ × 1″)	1 oz.	105	Grated	1 T.	30
Brick			Roquefort	1 oz.	105
(7⅛ × 3¾ × 3/32″)	1 oz.	105	Swiss		
Camembert (triangle			(3½ × 3⅜ × ⅛″)	1 oz.	100
sides: 2⅛″, 1⅛″ thick)	1 oz.	85	Cheese spreads	per oz.	85
Cheddar:			Cheese spreads	1 T.	40
Cylindrical,			Cream:		
Longhorn style			Cream substitute,		
(slice: 2⅝″ diam.,			non-dairy	1 T.	35
3⅝″ high)	9/10 oz.	95	Half-and-half	1 T.	20
Rectangular (slice:			Half-and-half	1 oz.	40
1¾ × 1⅝ × ¼″)	½ oz.	50	Light, coffee or table	1 T.	30
Round, midget			Light, coffee or table	1 oz.	60
Longhorn (slice:			Sour	½ cup	225
3¼″ diam., ⅛″ thick)	¾ oz.	85	Whipping, heavy	1 T.	55
Semicircular Longhorn			Whipping, heavy	1 oz.	100
(5⅝ × 3½ × ⅛″)	1¼ oz.	140	Whipping, light	1 T.	45
Shredded	¼ cup		Whipping, light	1 oz.	85
	(1 oz.)	115	Eggs (chicken):		
Squares (⅞ × ¾ × ½″)	⅕ oz.	20	Cooked		
Cottage	1 cup		(medium size):		
	(8 oz.)	240	Boiled	1	75
Cream	1 T.	52	Coddled	1	75
Edam	1 oz.	105	Deviled	2 halves	125
Fontina	1 oz.	115	Fried	1	100
Gorgonzola	1 oz.	110	Omelet	1	100
Gouda	1 oz.	110			
Gruyère	1 oz.	110			

ENERGY INTAKE TABLE, Continued

	Typical Measure	Calories (Rounded)		Typical Measure	Calories (Rounded)
Dairy Products, Cont.			Milk drinks, cont.:		
			Ice cream sodas, all		
Eggs, cooked, cont.:			flavors (1 scoop		
Poached	1	75	ice cream)	8 fluid oz.	175
Scrambled	2	200	Malted milk,		
Scrambled			all flavors	8 fluid oz.	225
with milk	2	250	Milk shakes,		
Shirred	1	75	all flavors	8 fluid oz.	200
Raw:			Yogurt, all flavors	1 cup	260
Large, white only	1	20	Yogurt, plain:		
Large, whole	1	90	With partially		
Large, yolk only	1	70	skimmed milk	1 cup	115
Small, white only	1	15	With whole milk	1 cup	140
Small, whole	1	65			
Small, yolk only	1	50			
Ice cream (all flavors):					
Regular, 10% fat	1 scoop°	65	**Desserts and Sweet Snacks**		
Regular, 12% fat	1 scoop	70	Cakes:		
Rich, 16% fat	1 scoop	80	Angel food	2 oz. slice	160
Ice milk	1 scoop	50	(2½" arc, 4" high)		
Sherbet	1 scoop	65	Boston cream	2½ oz.	
Frozen custard	1 scoop	85	(2⅛" arc, 3½" high)	slice	210
Milk:			Caramel	2¾ oz.	
Buttermilk	8 oz.	90	(1¾" arc, 3" high)	slice	300
Condensed,			Chocolate	3¹⁄₁₀ oz.	
sweetened	1 T.	65	(3 × 3 × 2")	slice	325
Dry, powdered	1 T.	35	Cupcake		
Evaporated,			(2¾" diam.)	⅕ oz.	120
unsweetened	1 T.	20	Fruitcake:		
Low-fat	8 oz.	130	Slice from loaf		
Non-fat	8 oz.	90	(¼ × 2 × 1½")	½ oz.	60
Skimmed	8 oz.	90	Wedge from tube		
Whole	8 oz.	160	(⅔" arc, 2¼" high)	1½ oz.	165
Milk drinks:			Gingerbread		
Chocolate milk	8 fluid oz.	210	(3 × 3 × 2")	4⅙ oz.	375
			Plain cake or cupcake:		
° 1 scoop = 2 fluid ounces. Sugar cone = 40 Cal.; Waffle cone = 20 Cal.			With boiled white icing (3 × 3 × 2")	4 oz.	400

	Typical Measure	Calories (Rounded)		Typical Measure	Calories (Rounded)
Cake, white icing, cont.:			Candies:°		
Cupcake			Butterscotch	1 oz.	115
(2½″ diam.)	1⅙ oz.	115	Candied fruits	1 oz.	90
Cupcake			Caramels	1 oz.	115
(2¾″ diam.)	1½ oz.	155	Caramels with nuts	1 oz.	120
With chocolate icing			Chocolate-flavored		
(3 × 3 × 2″)	4⅓ oz.	455	roll:		
Cupcake			4⅜″ long	1⅒ oz.	130
(2½″ diam.)	1¼ oz.	135	2½″ long	¼ oz.	30
Cupcake			Chocolate:		
(2¾″ diam.)	1⅔ oz.	175	Bittersweet	1 oz.	135
With uncooked white			Semisweet	1 oz.	145
icing (3 × 3 × 2″)	4¼ oz.	445	Sweet	1 oz.	150
Cupcake			Chocolate, milk	1 oz.	150
(2½″ diam.)	1¼ oz.	130	With almonds	1 oz.	150
Cupcake			With peanuts	1 oz.	155
(2¾″ diam.)	1⅔ oz.	175	Chocolate coated:		
Without icing			Almonds	1 oz.	160
(3 × 3 × 2″)	3 oz.	315	Chocolate fudge	1 oz.	125
Cupcake			Chocolate fudge		
(2½″ diam.)	9/10 oz.	90	with nuts	1 oz.	130
Cupcake			Coconut center	1 oz.	125
(2¾″ diam.)	1⅙ oz.	120	Fondant:		
Pound (slice from loaf			Mints, round:		
3½ × 3 × ½″)	1 oz.	145	Large (2½″ diam.,		
Sponge			⅜″ thick)	1¼ oz.	145
(2½″ arc, 4″ high)	2⅓ oz.	195	Miniature		
White (2-layer):			(¾″ diam., ⅜″ thick)	1/10 oz.	10
With coconut icing			Small (1⅜″ diam.,		
(2⅜″ arc, 3″ high)	3⅔ oz.	390	⅜″ thick)	⅖ oz.	45
With uncooked			Fudge, caramel,		
white icing			peanuts	1 oz.	125
(2⅛″ arc, 3″ high)	2 9/10 oz.	310	Honeycombed		
Yellow:			hard candy,		
With caramel icing			peanut butter	1 oz.	130
(2⅜″ arc, 3″ high)	3 9/10 oz.	390			
With chocolate					
icing (2⅜″ arc, 3″ high)	3½ oz.	365			

° Typical measure, fine candies: 1 piece = ± 1 oz. Wrapped candy bars usually will weigh between 1 and 2 oz. Weight and contents on label.

ENERGY INTAKE TABLE, Continued

	Typical Measure	Calories (Rounded)		Typical Measure	Calories (Rounded)
Desserts and Sweet Snacks, Cont.			Candies, cont.:		
			Taffy, chocolate-		
Candies, cont.:°			flavored	1 oz.	110
Nougat and			Toffee	1 oz.	110
caramel	1 oz.	120	Cookies (*quantity:* size):		
Peanuts (single			Assorted (3)	per oz.	135
nuts, 8 to 16;			Brownies with nuts		
clusters, 2)	1 oz.	160	(*1:* 3 × 1 × ⅞″)	¾ oz.	100
Raisins (single,			Butter (5 or 6:		
18 to 28;			2″ diam., ¼″ thick)	1 oz.	130
clusters, 2)	1 oz.	120	Chocolate chip (3:		
Vanilla creams	1 oz.	125	2⅓″ diam.)	1 oz.	150
Fondant, uncoated	1 oz.	105	Chocolate snaps (4:		
Fudge:			2″ diam., ¼″ thick)	1 oz.	135
Chocolate or			Coconut bars (3:		
vanilla	1 oz.	115	2⅜ × 1⅝ × ⅜″)	1 oz.	150
With nuts	1 oz.	120	Fig bars (2:		
Gumdrops	1 oz.	100	1½ × 1¾ × ½″)	1 oz.	100
Hard	1 oz.	110	Gingersnaps (4:		
Jellybeans (10 beans:			2″ diam., ¼″ thick)	1 oz.	120
¾″ long)	1 oz.	105	Ladyfingers (2½:		
Marshmallows:			3¼ × 1⅜ × 1⅛″,		
All sizes	per oz.	90	before split)	1 oz.	105
Large (1⅛″ diam.,			Macaroons (2:		
¾″ high)	each	25	2¾″ diam., ¼″ thick)	1⅓ oz.	185
Miniature			Marshmallow:		
(½″ diam., ½″ high)	1 cup	150	Chocolate-coated (2:		
Peanut bars	per oz.	145	1¾″ diam., ¾″ thick)	1 oz.	110
Peanut brittle	per oz.	120	Coconut-coated (2:		
Sugar-coated almonds			2⅛″ diam., 1⅛″ thick)	1 oz.	150
(8)	per oz.	130	Molasses (1:		
Sugar-coated			3⅝″ diam., ¾″ thick)	1(+) oz.	140
chocolate disks			Oatmeal (2:		
(31 disks: ½″ diam.)	per oz.	135	2⅝″ diam., ¼″ thick)	1 oz.	130
Taffy, all flavors			Peanut:		
except chocolate	1 oz.	105	Sandwich type (2:		
			1¾″ diam., ½″ thick)	9/10 oz.	115
			Sugar wafer (4:		
			1¾ × 1⅜ × ⅜″)	1 oz.	135

° Typical measure, fine candies: 1 piece = ± 1 oz. Wrapped candy bars usually will weigh between 1 and 2 oz. Weight and contents on label.

	Typical Measure	Calories (Rounded)		Typical Measure	Calories (Rounded)
Cookies, cont.:			French pastries (see		
Raisin (2:			Pastries and Tarts)		
$2\frac{1}{4} \times 2\frac{1}{2} \times \frac{1}{4}''$)	$1\frac{1}{4}$ oz.	135	Fritters, apple or banana		
Sandwich, chocolate or			(2″ diam., 2″ thick)	$1\frac{1}{2}$ oz.	200
vanilla:			Fruits (see separate		
Oval (2:			listing of Fruits)		
$3\frac{1}{8} \times 1\frac{1}{4} \times \frac{3}{8}''$)	1 oz.	150	Gelatin	$\frac{1}{2}$ cup	70
Round (3:			Gum, chewing	per stick	10
$1\frac{3}{4}''$ diam., $\frac{3}{8}''$ thick)	1 oz.	150	Pastries and tarts:		
Shortbread (4:			Cream puffs, custard		
$1\frac{5}{8} \times 1\frac{5}{8} \times \frac{1}{4}''$)	1 oz.	140	filling ($3\frac{1}{2}''$ diam.,		
Sugar (3:			2″ high)	$4\frac{1}{2}$ oz.	300
$2\frac{1}{4}''$ diam., $\frac{1}{4}''$ thick)	$\frac{9}{10}$ oz.	110	Eclairs, custard filling,		
Sugar wafers (3:			chocolate icing		
$3\frac{1}{2} \times 1 \times \frac{1}{2}''$)	1(+) oz.	135	(5 × 2 × $1\frac{3}{4}''$)	$3\frac{1}{2}$ oz.	240
Vanilla wafers (7:			French pastries,		
$1\frac{3}{4}''$ diam., $\frac{1}{4}''$ thick)	1 oz.	130	assorted	per oz.	150
Dessert toppings:			Pies°:		
Butterscotch	1 T.	60	Apple	$5\frac{1}{2}$ oz.	405
Caramel	1 T.	60	Diet slice	1(+) oz.	85
Chocolate,			Banana custard	$5\frac{1}{3}$ oz.	335
bittersweet	1 T.	70	Diet slice	1(+) oz.	70
Chocolate, fudge	1 T.	60	Blackberry	$5\frac{1}{2}$ oz.	385
Chocolate, milk	1 T.	75	Diet slice	1(+) oz.	80
Custard	1 T.	11	Blueberry	$5\frac{1}{3}$ oz.	385
Hard sauce, heavy	1 T.	100	Diet slice	1(+) oz.	80
Marshmallow	1 T.	45	Boston cream (see		
Mint	1 T.	55	Cakes)		
Nut	1 T.	65	Butterscotch	$5\frac{1}{3}$ oz.	405
Pineapple	1 T.	40	Diet slice	1(+) oz.	85
Strawberry	1 T.	40	Cherry	$5\frac{1}{2}$ oz.	410
Whipped	1 T.	15	Diet slice	$1\frac{1}{5}$ oz.	90
Doughnuts:			Chocolate chiffon	4(−) oz.	355
Cake, large (1:			Diet slice	$\frac{4}{5}$ oz.	75
$3\frac{3}{8}''$ diam., $1\frac{1}{4}''$ high)	2 oz.	225	Chocolate meringue	$5\frac{1}{3}$ oz.	385
Cake, small (1:			Diet slice	1(+) oz.	80
$1\frac{1}{2}''$ diam., $\frac{3}{4}''$ high)	$\frac{1}{2}$ oz.	55			
Yeast leavened (1:					
$3\frac{3}{4}''$ diam., $1\frac{1}{4}''$ high)	$1\frac{1}{4}$ oz.	175			

° Regular slices are $\frac{1}{6}$ of pie, 9″ diam. Arc of slice is $4\frac{3}{4}''$. Diet slice has 1″ arc.

ENERGY INTAKE TABLE, Continued

	Typical Measure	Calories (Rounded)		Typical Measure	Calories (Rounded)
Desserts and Sweet Snacks, Cont.			Puddings, cont.:		
			Banana	½ cup (3¾ oz.)	165
Pies, cont.:°					
Coconut custard	5⅓ oz.	360	Bread, with raisins	½ cup (4⅔ oz.)	250
Diet slice	1(+) oz.	75			
Custard	5⅓ oz.	330	Butterscotch	½ cup (4½ oz.)	160
Diet slice	1(+) oz.	70			
Lemon chiffon	4(−) oz.	340	Chocolate	½ cup (4½ oz.)	165
Diet slice	⅘ oz.	70			
Lemon meringue	5(−) oz.	360	Custard, baked	½ cup (4⅔ oz.)	150
Diet slice	1 oz.	75			
Mince	5½ oz.	430	Indian	½ cup (4½ oz.)	125
Diet slice	1(+) oz.	90			
Peach	5⅓ oz.	405	Lemon	½ cup (4½ oz.)	150
Diet slice	1(+) oz.	85			
Pecan	5(−) oz.	580	Plum	½ cup (4½ oz.)	150
Diet slice	1 oz.	125			
Pineapple	5½ oz.	400	Rice, with raisins	½ cup (4⅔ oz.)	195
Diet slice	1(+) oz.	85			
Pineapple chiffon	4(−) oz.	310	Tapioca	½ cup (3 oz.)	110
Diet slice	⅘ oz.	65			
Pineapple custard	5⅓ oz.	335	Vanilla	½ cup (4½ oz.)	150
Diet slice	1(+) oz.	70			
Pumpkin	5⅓ oz.	320			
Diet slice	1(+) oz.	70	**Fats and Oils**		
Raisin	5½ oz.	430	Butter	1 T.	100
Diet slice	1(+) oz.	90	Cooking oils, animal or		
Rhubarb	5½ oz.	400	vegetable	1 T.	120
Diet slice	1(+) oz.	85	Margarine	1 T.	100
Strawberry	4⅓ oz.	250	Lard	1 T.	117
Diet slice	1(−) oz.	55			
Sweet potato	5⅓ oz.	325	**Fruit (_quantity:_ size)**		
Diet slice	1(+) oz.	70			
Puddings:			Acerola (_10:_ 1″ diam.)	3½ oz.	25
Apple brown betty	½ cup (3¾ oz.)	165	Apple, large (3¼″ diam.)	8 oz.	125
			Small (2½″ diam.)	4 oz.	60
			Applesauce, sweetened (½ cup)	4½ oz.	120
			Unsweetened (½ cup)	4⅓ oz.	50

° Regular slices are ⅙ of pie, 9″ diam. Arc of slice is 4¾″. Diet slice has 1″ arc.

	Typical Measure	Calories (Rounded)		Typical Measure	Calories (Rounded)
Apricots (3)	4 oz.	55	Dates, cont.:		
Avocados (½ of 3⅛" diam.)	4½ oz.	190	Chopped (½ cup)	3 oz.	245
Bananas:			Elderberries (1 cup)	3½ oz.	75
Large (9¾" long,			Figs:		
1⁷⁄₁₆" diam.)	7 oz.	115	Large (2½" diam.)	2¼ oz.	55
Medium (8¾" long,			Medium (2¼" diam.)	1¾ oz.	40
1⅜" diam.)	6 oz.	100	Small (1½" diam.)	1⅖ oz.	35
Small (7¾" long,			Fruit cocktail or salad,		
1⅜" diam.)	5 oz.	90	syrup (½ cup)	4½ oz.	100
Blackberries (1 cup)	5 oz.	85	Fruit cocktail or salad,		
Blueberries (1 cup)	5 oz.	90	water pack (½ cup)	4⅓ oz.	45
Boysenberries, canned			Gooseberries (1 cup)	5¼ oz.	60
(1 cup)	9 oz.	90	Grapefruit (½ of		
Breadfruit, fresh, peeled			4" diam.)	6½ oz.	40
(1)	4 oz.	120	Cut-up sections		
Cantaloupe			(1 cup)	8 oz.	95
(½ of 5" diam.)	8½ oz.	80	Grapes:		
Casaba (1⁄10 of melon			American° (10:		
wedge, 7¾" long,			¾" diam.)	1⅖ oz.	20
2" wide)	8½ oz.	40	European° (10:		
Cherries:			⅝" to ¾" diam.)	2 oz.	40
Raw, whole (with pits			Guava (1)	3½ oz.	65
and stems):			Honeydew melon (1⁄10		
Candied (10)	1¼ oz.	120	wedge: 7" long, 2" wide)	8 oz.	50
Sour, red (1 cup)	4 oz.	60	Jujube, dried	4 oz.	300
Sweet (10)	2½ oz.	50	Fresh	4 oz.	110
Canned (pitted,			Kumquats (1)	⅔ oz.	15
water pack):			Lemons (2¼" diam.)	4½ oz.	25
Sour (1 cup)	8½ oz.	105	Peel, grated	1 T.	0
Sweet (1 cup)	9 oz.	210	Wedge (1¼" arc)	1(−) oz.	5
Cherries, West Indian			Limes (2" diam.)	3(−) oz.	20
(10: 1" diam.)	3½ oz.	25	Litchi nuts, dried,		
Crabapples (1)	3½ oz.	70	shelled (10)	5 oz.	70
Cranberries (1 cup)	3⅓ oz.	45	Loganberries (1 cup)	5 oz.	90
Cranberry sauce,			Loquats (10)	5½ oz.	60
sweetened (½ cup)	5 oz.	200			
Currants, black, red or					
white (1 cup)	4 oz.	65			
Dates (10)	3 oz.	220			

° American grapes: Concord, Delaware, Niagara, Catawba, Scuppernong. European: Thompson seedless, Emperor, Flame Tokay, Ribier, Malaga, Muscat.

ENERGY INTAKE TABLE, Continued

	Typical Measure	Calories (Rounded)		Typical Measure	Calories (Rounded)
Fruit, Cont.			Pineapple, cont.:		
			Canned, water pack		
Mangos, diced or sliced			(½ cup)	4⅓ oz.	50
(1 cup)	6(−) oz.	110	Fresh (1 slice:		
Melon balls in syrup			3½" diam., ¾" thick)	3 oz.	45
(1 cup)	8 oz.	145	Pomegranate (1:		
Mulberries (1 cup)	4 oz.	85	3⅜" diam., 2¾" high)	9¾ oz.	100
Nectarines (2½" diam.)	5¼ oz.	90	Prunes (4)	1¾ oz.	110
Oranges (2⅝" diam.)	6⅓ oz.	65	Pumpkin (½ cup)	4⅓ oz.	40
Cut up sections			Quince (1: 3" diam.)	3½ oz.	55
(1 cup)	5½ oz.	80	Raisins (⅓ cup)	1½ oz.	125
Large (3+" diam.)	9 oz.	95	Raspberries:	1 T.	25
Peel, grated	1 oz.	0	Black (1 cup)	4¾ oz.	100
Wedge (2" arc)	1(+) oz.	15	Red (1 cup)	4⅓ oz.	70
Papaw (1: 3¾" long,			Rhubarb, cooked,		
2" diam.)	4½ oz.	85	sweetened (½ cup)	4¾ oz.	190
Papaya (1: 5⅛" high,			Strawberries (1 cup)	5¼ oz.	55
3½" diam.)	16 oz.	120	Tangerines (2½" diam.)	4 oz.	40
Passion fruit (Granadilla)			Sections (1 cup)	6¾ oz.	90
(1)	1¼ oz.	15	Watermelon (4" arc:		
Peaches:			8" radius or		
Canned, syrup pack			10" diam., 1" thick)	32 oz.	110
(1 half)	2¾ oz.	60	Diced pieces (1 cup)	8+ oz.	45
Canned, water pack					
(1 half)	2¾ oz.	25			
Large (1: 2¾" diam.)	6⅕ oz.	60	**Meat, Fish and Game°**		
Small (1: 2½" diam.)	4 oz.	40	Summary:°°		
Pears (1: 2½" diam.,			Animal organs	per oz.	41
3½" high)	6⅓ oz.	100	Beef, lean	per oz.	78
Canned, syrup pack			Fish	per oz.	38
(1 half)	3½ oz.	80	Fowl	per oz.	41
Canned, water pack			Lamb, lean	per oz.	78
(1 half)	2¾ oz.	25	Pork, lean	per oz.	91
Persimmons:			Shellfish	per oz.	30
Japanese			Veal, lean	per oz.	63
(2½" diam., 3" high)	7 oz.	130			
Native	1 oz.	30			
Pineapple:					
Canned, syrup pack					
(½ cup)	4½ oz.	95			

° Edible portions only. Weights before cooking unless otherwise specified.

°° For handy reference, particularly when specific detail is not known.

	Typical Measure	Calories (Rounded)		Typical Measure	Calories (Rounded)
Fish and Shellfish*			Fish cakes (*1:* 3″ diam., ½″ thick)	2(+) oz.	105
Abalone, 1 steak	4 oz.	110	Fish sticks (4 × 1 × ½″)	1 oz.	50
Albacore	4 oz.	200	Flounder, baked with		
Anchovies, canned,			butter or margarine (1		
pickled (5 fillets)	⅔ oz.	35	fillet: 8¼ × 2¾ × ¼″)	3½ oz.	200
Bass, black sea, baked,			Grouper	4 oz.	100
stuffed (3½ × 4½ × 1½″)	7¼ oz.	530	Haddock, fried (fillet:		
Bass, striped, oven fried			6⅜ × 2½ × ⅝″)	4 oz.	185
(8¾ × 4½ × ⅝″)	7 oz.	395	Halibut, broiled with		
Bluefish:			butter (fillet:		
Baked or broiled			6½ × 2 × ⅝″)	4½ oz.	215
(1 fillet: 7¾ × 3⅞ × ⅜″)	5½ oz.	250	Herring, plain	per oz.	60
Fried (1 fillet:			In tomato sauce		
8⅛ × 3¼ × ¾″)	6¾ oz.	400	(4¾ × 1⅛ × ⅝″)	2 oz.	100
Bonito	4 oz.	190	Pickled		
Carp	4 oz.	130	(7 × 1½ × ½″)	1½ oz.	115
Catfish	4 oz.	120	Smoked, kippered		
Caviar, granular	1 T.	42	(7 × 2¼ × ¼″)	2¼ oz.	140
Pressed	1 T.	54	Lobster	per oz.	27
Pressed	per oz.	90	Newburg (1 cup)	9 oz.	485
Chub	4 oz.	165	Salad (½ cup)	4 oz.	285
Clam fritters (*1:*			Mackerel:		
2″ diam., 1¾″ thick)	1⅖ oz.	125	Atlantic (fillet:		
Clams (4 cherrystones or			8½ × 2½ × ½″)	3½ oz.	250
5 littlenecks)	2½ oz.	55	Pacific	3½ oz.	180
Cod, fillet, broiled			Salted (fillet:		
(5 × 2½ × ⅞″)	2¼ oz.	110	7¾ × 2½ × ½″)	4 oz.	340
Crab:	per oz.	27	Mullet	4 oz.	170
Blue, Dungeness,			Mussels	per oz.	27
rock, king (1 cup)	5½ oz.	145	Ocean perch, fried		
Crayfish	4 oz.	110	(fillet: 6¾ × 1¾ × ⅝″)	3 oz.	280
Eel:	4 oz.	265	Octopus	per oz.	21
Smoked	4 oz.	375	Oysters:		
Finnan haddie	4 oz.	120	Eastern (2 to 3)	1 oz.	20
			Pacific (4 to 6)	8½ oz.	220
			Fried (2 to 3)	1 oz.	70
			Perch, white	4 oz.	135
* Edible portions only. Weights before cooking unless otherwise specified.			Perch, yellow	4 oz.	100
			Pike	4 oz.	100

ENERGY INTAKE TABLE, Continued

	Typical Measure	Calories (Rounded)		Typical Measure	Calories (Rounded)
Fish and Shellfish, Cont.°			Beef°°:		
			Brisket, braised		
Pollock, cooked,			($4\frac{1}{8} \times 2\frac{1}{4} \times \frac{1}{2}''$)	3 oz.	190
creamed	4 oz.	145	Chuck, ground		
Pompano	4 oz.	190	($3''$ diam., $\frac{5}{8}''$ thick)	3 oz.	185
Red and gray snapper	4 oz.	110	Chuck rib roast		
Salmon, broiled or baked			($4\frac{1}{8} \times 2\frac{1}{4} \times \frac{1}{2}''$)	3 oz.	215
with butter	4 oz.	210	Chuck roast, arm and		
Salmon, smoked	4 oz.	200	round bone cuts		
Sardines	per oz.	90	($2\frac{1}{2} \times 2\frac{1}{2} \times \frac{3}{4}''$)	3 oz.	165
Scallops, fried (10 to 15)	4 oz.	210	Club steak	7 oz.	470
Shrimp:			Corned beef (3 slices:		
Large (*10: 3¼'' long*)	2 oz.	70	$3 \times 2 \times \frac{3}{8}''$)	4 oz.	315
Medium (*10: 2½'' long*)	1(+) oz.	40	Corned beef hash	1 cup	400
Small (*10: 2'' long*)	$\frac{3}{5}$ oz.	20	Dried, chipped,		
Sole	4 oz.	230	creamed	1 cup	375
Squid	per oz.	24	Filet mignon	4 oz.	335
Sturgeon, smoked	4 oz.	170	Flank steak		
Swordfish	4 oz.	135	($2\frac{1}{2} \times 2\frac{1}{2} \times \frac{3}{4}''$)	3 oz.	165
Trout, brook	4 oz.	120	Ground round		
Trout, rainbow	4 oz.	200	($3''$ diam., $\frac{5}{8}''$ thick)	3 oz.	185
Tuna:			Hamburger		
Raw (2 T.)	per oz.	40	($3''$ diam., $\frac{5}{8}''$ thick)	3 oz.	185
Packed in oil, drained			Porterhouse steak	6 oz.	385
solids	per oz.	55	Pot pie		
Packed in water	per oz.	35	($\frac{1}{6}$ of $9''$ diameter pie)	$3\frac{3}{4}$ oz.	260
Salad	per oz.	50	Pot roast	4 oz.	330
Salad	$\frac{1}{2}$ cup	200	Rib roast		
			($4\frac{1}{8} \times 2\frac{1}{4} \times \frac{1}{4}''$)	3 oz.	205
			Round steak		
Meat and Game°			($4\frac{1}{8} \times 2\frac{1}{4} \times \frac{1}{2}''$)	3 oz.	160
Bacon, Canadian			Rump roast		
($3\frac{3}{8}''$ diam., $\frac{3}{16}''$ thick)	$\frac{3}{4}$ oz.	6	($4\frac{1}{8} \times 2\frac{1}{4} \times \frac{1}{4}''$)	3 oz.	180
Bacon, crisp			Sirloin steak,		
(medium strip)	$\frac{1}{2}$ oz.	50	double-bone	$7\frac{1}{2}$ oz.	475

° Calories are shown for weights, ready-to-cook, edible portions, unless otherwise specified.

°° Typical measures are choice grade (75% lean, 25% fat), lean cut, trimmed of separable fat, cooked, ready to serve.

	Typical Measure	Calories (Rounded)		Typical Measure	Calories (Rounded)
Beef, cont.:			Chicken, cont.:		
Sirloin steak, double-bone (2½ × 2½ × ¾″)	3 oz.	185	Fryers, fried: Dark meat, without skin (11 pieces: 1⅞ × 2 × ¼″)	4 oz.	250
Sirloin steak, hip bone	6½ oz.	450	Light meat, without skin (4½ pieces:		
Sirloin steak, hip bone (2½ × 2½ × ¾″)	3 oz.	205	2½ × 1⅞ × ¼″)	4 oz.	225
Sirloin steak, round bone	7½ oz.	450	Cut-up parts from 2½ lb. fryer:		
Sirloin steak, round bone (3½ × 2 × ¾″)	3 oz.	175	Back (67% edible)	2(+) oz.	140
Stew with vegetables	1 cup	220	Breast (84% edible)	6¾ oz.	320
T-bone steak	6 oz.	375	Drumstick (67% edible)	2(−) oz.	90
Chicken:			Neck (73% edible)	2(+) oz.	130
Baked or roasted (all classes):			Rib section (69% edible), 2 halves	1⅖ oz.	85
Dark meat, without skin (11 pieces:			Thigh (79% edible)	2⅓ oz.	125
1⅞ × 1 × ¼″)	4 oz.	200	Wing (61% edible)	1¾ oz.	85
Light meat, without skin (4½ pieces:			Giblets (1 cup), fried	5(+) oz.	360
2½ × 1⅞ × ¼″)	4 oz.	190	Livers (1: 2 × 2 × ⅝″)	1(−) oz.	40
Boiled or stewed (hens and cocks):			Livers, chopped (1 cup), cooked	5 oz.	230
Dark meat, without skin (11 pieces:			Pot pie (about ⅙ of 9″ diam. pie)	4 oz.	265
1⅞ × 1 × ¼″)	4 oz.	235	Duck, roasted (3 pieces: 3½ × 2½ × ¼″)	3½ oz.	325
Light meat without skin (4½ pieces:			Frogs' legs, fried (2)	1½ oz.	150
2½ × 1⅞ × ¼″)	4 oz.	205	Goat meat	4 oz.	200
Broilers, broiled (½ broiler, 60% edible)	10½ oz.	240	Goose, roasted (2½ pieces: 3½ × 3 × ¼″)	3 oz.	200
Canned, boned (½ of 5½ oz. can)	2¾ oz.	155	Guinea hen	3½ oz.	160
Chicken à la king (scant ½ cup)	4 oz.	215	Ham:		
Fricassee, cooked (scant ½ cup)	4 oz.	185	Baked or roasted: Lean with fat (2 pieces: 4⅛ × 2¼ × ¼″)	3 oz.	320

ENERGY INTAKE TABLE, Continued

	Typical Measure	Calories (Rounded)		Typical Measure	Calories (Rounded)
Meat and Game, Cont. *			Lamb shoulder, cont.:		
			Lean with fat		
Ham, baked, cont.:			(74% lean, 26% fat)	3 oz.	290
Lean, trimmed of			Lean, trimmed of		
separable fat			separable fat	3 oz.	175
(2 pieces:			Liver (fried, simmered		
$4\frac{1}{8} \times 2\frac{1}{4} \times \frac{1}{4}''$)	3 oz.	185	or broiled):		
Boiled (1 slice:			Beef (1 slice:		
$4\frac{1}{4}''$ diam., $\frac{1}{16}''$ thick)	$\frac{3}{4}$ oz.	50	$6\frac{1}{2} \times 2\frac{3}{8} \times \frac{3}{8}''$)	3 oz.	195
Canned (cured)	4 oz.	220	Calf (1 slice:		
Deviled, canned	1 oz.	100	$6\frac{1}{2} \times 2\frac{3}{8} \times \frac{3}{8}''$)	3 oz.	225
Deviled, canned	1 T.	45	Chicken (1 liver:	less than	
Croquette (1" diam.,			$2 \times 2 \times \frac{5}{8}''$)	1 oz.	40
3" long)	each	165	Chicken, chopped		
Lamb:			(1 cup)	5 oz.	230
Leg (2 pieces, roasted:			Hog (1 slice:		
$4\frac{1}{8} \times 2\frac{1}{4} \times \frac{1}{4}''$)			$6\frac{1}{2} \times 2\frac{3}{8} \times \frac{3}{8}''$)	3 oz.	205
Lean with fat			Lamb (1 slice:		
(83% lean, 17% fat)	3 oz.	240	$3\frac{1}{2} \times 2 \times \frac{3}{8}''$)	$1\frac{3}{5}$ oz.	120
Lean, trimmed of			Turkey, chopped		
separable fat	3 oz.	160	(1 cup)	5 oz.	245
Loin chops, broiled			Liver paste	per oz.	130
(cut 3 per pound):			Pate de foie gras	1 T.	60
Lean with fat			Pheasant	4 oz.	150
(66% lean, 34% fat)	$3\frac{2}{5}$ oz.	340	Pigs feet, pickled	per oz.	60
Lean, trimmed of			Pork:		
separable fat	$2\frac{1}{3}$ oz.	125	Baked or roasted loin		
Rib chops, broiled			roast (1 piece:		
(cut 3 per pound):			$2\frac{1}{2} \times 2\frac{1}{2} \times \frac{3}{4}''$):		
Lean with fat			Lean, trimmed of		
(62% lean, 38% fat)	3 oz.	365	separable fat	3 oz.	215
Lean, trimmed of			Lean with fat		
separable fat	2 oz.	120	(80% lean, 20% fat)	3 oz.	310
Shoulder (3 pieces:			Broiled loin chops:		
$2\frac{1}{2} \times 2\frac{1}{2} \times \frac{1}{4}''$),			Lean, trimmed of		
roasted:			separable fat	2 oz.	150
			Lean with fat		
			(72% lean, 28% fat)	$2\frac{7}{10}$ oz.	305

* Calories are shown for weights, ready-to-cook, edible portions, unless otherwise specified.

	Typical Measure	Calories (Rounded)		Typical Measure	Calories (Rounded)
Pork, cont.:			Sausages, cold cuts and		
Shoulder cuts:			luncheon meats, cont.:		
Boston butt, roasted			Cervelat (4 slices:	less than	
(3 pieces:			1½″ diam., ⅛″ thick)	½ oz.)	55
2½ × 2½ × ¼″):			Deviled ham, canned	1 oz.	100
Lean, trimmed of			Frankfurter		
separable fat	3 oz.	210	(5″ long, ⅞″ thick)	2 oz.	175
Lean with fat			Headcheese		
(79% lean, 21% fat)	3 oz.	300	(4 × 4 × ³⁄₃₂″ thick)	1 oz.	75
Picnic, simmered			Knockwurst (1 link:		
(3 pieces:			4″ long, 1⅛″ diam.)	2½ oz.	190
2½ × 2½ × ¼″):			Liverwurst	2 oz.	175
Lean, trimmed of			Luncheon meat:		
separable fat	3 oz.	180	Boiled ham	¾ oz.	
Lean with fat			(4¼ × 4¼ × ¹⁄₁₆″)	per slice	50
(74% lean, 26% fat)	3 oz.	320	Chopped or spiced		
Spareribs, lean with			pork	per oz.	85
fat, braised	3 oz.	375	Meat loaf	per oz.	60
Spareribs, lean with			Meat, potted	per oz.	70
fat, braised	per oz.	125	Mortadella		
Quail	per oz.	50	(4⅞″ diam., ³⁄₃₂″ thick)	per oz.	90
Rabbit, stewed or baked	3 oz.	185	Polish sausage		
Sausages, cold cuts and			(5⅜″ long, 1″ diam.)	2¾ oz.	230
luncheon meats:			Pork sausage, cooked:		
Blood sausage (slice:			Link (4″ long,		
2¼″ diam., ⅛″ thick)	¼(+) oz.	32	⅞″ thick)	1 oz.	60
Bockwurst (1 link)	2⅓ oz.	175	Patty (3⅞″ diam.,		
Bologna (4½″ diam.)	1 oz.	85	¼″ thick)	2 oz.	130
Braunschweiger			Salami, dry	per oz.	130
(3 slices:			Large slice		
2″ diam., ¼″ thick)	1 oz.	95	(3⅛″ diam., ¹⁄₁₆″ thick)	⅓ oz.	45
Brown and serve, link	less than		Small slice		
(3⅞″ long)	1 oz.	85	(1¾″ diam., ⅛″ thick)	⅙ oz.	25
Brown and serve,			Salami, cooked (slice:		
patty (oval:			4½″ diam.)	1 oz.	90
2⅜ × 1⅞, ½″ thick)	1 oz.	110	Scrapple (slice:		
Capicola (slice:	less than		2¾″ × 2⅛″ × ¼″)	1 oz.	60
4¼ × 4¼ × ¹⁄₁₆″)	1 oz.	105			

ENERGY INTAKE TABLE, Continued

	Typical Measure	Calories (Rounded)		Typical Measure	Calories (Rounded)
Meat and Game, Cont.[*]			Veal, cont.:		
			Loin, braised, broiled		
Sausages, cold cuts and			(1 piece:		
luncheon meats, cont.:			$2\frac{1}{2} \times 2\frac{1}{2} \times \frac{3}{4}''$)	3 oz.	200
Thuringer cervelat			Plate, breast		
(slice: $4\frac{3}{8}''$ diam.,			(braised or stewed)	3 oz.	260
$\frac{1}{8}''$ thick)	1 oz.	90	Rib, roasted (2 pieces:		
Vienna sausage, canned			$4\frac{1}{8} \times 2\frac{1}{4} \times \frac{1}{4}''$)	3 oz.	230
(2" long, $\frac{7}{8}''$ diam.)	$\frac{1}{2}$ oz.	40	Round with rump,		
Sweetbreads, braised:			braised or broiled:		
Beef (yearlings)	3 oz.	275	Cutlets (1 piece:		
Calf	3 oz.	145	$4\frac{1}{8} \times 2\frac{1}{4} \times \frac{1}{2}''$)	3 oz.	185
Lamb	3 oz.	150	Roasts (2 pieces:		
Tongue, braised			$4\frac{1}{8} \times 2\frac{1}{4} \times \frac{1}{4}''$)	3 oz.	185
($3 \times 2 \times \frac{1}{8}''$):			Venison, lean	3 oz.	110
Beef	$\frac{2}{3}$ oz.	50			
Calves'	$\frac{2}{3}$ oz.	35			
Hog	$\frac{2}{3}$ oz.	50	**Miscellaneous (Cooking Measures, Flour,**		
Lamb	$\frac{2}{3}$ oz.	50	**Pastas, etc.)**		
Sheep	$\frac{2}{3}$ oz.	65	Arrowroot	1 T.	30
Turkey, roasted, without			Baking powders:		
skin:			Sodium aluminum		
Canned ($\frac{1}{2}$ cup)	$3\frac{1}{2}$ oz.	210	sulfate	1 T.	14
Dark meat (4 pieces:			Straight phosphate	1 T.	15
$2\frac{1}{2} \times 1\frac{5}{8} \times \frac{1}{4}''$)	3 oz.	175	Tartrate	1 T.	7
Giblets (1 cup)	5 oz.	340	Low-sodium		
Light meat (2 pieces:			preparations	1 T.	23
$4 \times 2 \times \frac{1}{4}''$)	3 oz.	150	Barley ($\frac{1}{2}$ cup, dry =		
Hash	1 cup	300	2 cups, cooked)	$3\frac{1}{2}$ oz.	350
Pot pie			Barley	1 T.	45
($\frac{1}{6}$ of pie, 9" diam.)	4 oz.	275	Bran (1 cup)	$2\frac{1}{10}$ oz.	145
Veal:			Buckwheat flour, dark		
Chuck, braised, pot-			(1 cup)	$3\frac{1}{2}$ oz.	325
roasted or stewed:			Buckwheat flour, light		
(1 piece:			(1 cup)	$3\frac{1}{2}$ oz.	340
$2\frac{1}{2} \times 2\frac{1}{2} \times \frac{3}{4}''$)	3 oz.	200	Bulgar ($\frac{1}{2}$ cup, dry =		
			$1\frac{1}{2}$ cup, cooked)	3(−) oz.	300
			Bulgar	1 T.	40
			Cheese fondue	per oz.	100

[*] Calories are shown for weights, ready-to-cook, edible portions, unless otherwise specified.

	Typical Measure	Calories (Rounded)		Typical Measure	Calories (Rounded)
Chili con carne, with beans (½ cup)	4½ oz.	170	Masa Harina (1 cup)	3⁹⁄₁₀ oz.	405
Chili con carne, without beans (½ cup)	5 oz.	200	Millet (⅓ cup, dry = 1 cup, cooked)	2 oz.	195
Chop suey, with meat (½ cup)	4⅖ oz.	150	Mustard, dry	1 t.	5
Chow mein, chicken (½ cup)	4⅖ oz.	130	Noodles (1 cup)	5⅔ oz.	200
Cocoa, dry	1 T.	15	Noodles, chow mein (1 cup)	1½ oz.	220
Coffee, dry	1 T.	5	Pastina, egg, dry (1 cup)	6 oz.	650
Coffee, dry°	1 t.	1	Pastina, egg, dry	1 T.	40
Coffee, liquid (1 cup)°	6½ oz.	2	Peanut butter	1 T.	95
Cooking oils, animal or vegetable	1 T.	120	Peanut flour, defatted (1 cup)	2 oz.	225
Corn flour (1 cup)	4¹⁄₁₀ oz.	430	Pimientos (glass jar, size 2Z)	2 oz.	15
Corn flour	1 T.	27	Pizza (14″ diam. pie):		
Corn meal, whole ground (1 cup, dry = 4 cups, cooked)	4⅓ oz.	435	Cheese (⅛ slice)	2¼ oz.	155
Degermed, dry (1 cup)	4⁹⁄₁₀ oz.	500	Sausage (⅛ slice)	2¼ oz.	160
Degermed, cooked (½ cup)	4¼ oz.	60	Popcorn, popped:		
Corn starch	1 T.	30	Plain	1 cup	25
Curry powder	1 t.	5	Sugar-coated	1 cup	135
Farina, dry (½ cup)	3⅓ oz.	345	With oil and salt	1 cup	40
Kasha (½ cup dry = 1 cup cooked)	3½ oz.	260	Potato flour (1 cup)	8 oz.	525
Lard	1 T.	117	Potato flour	1 T.	35
Macaroni, cooked (1 cup)	4½ oz.	195	Pretzels (for detailed listings *see* Appetizers and Snacks)	per oz.	110
Macaroni and cheese (1 cup)	8½ oz.	230	Rice, cooked:		
Maize (corn flour) (1 cup)	4¹⁄₁₀ oz.	430	Brown (½ cup)	3½ oz.	115
Malt, dry	1 oz.	105	Spanish (½ cup)	4⅓ oz.	105
Manioc flour (1 cup)	3½ oz.	360	White (½ cup)	3½ oz.	100
Manioc flour	1 T.	25	Wild rice (½ cup)	2 oz.	200
			Rice, uncooked (½ cup)	3½ oz.	355
			Rice, uncooked	1 T.	45
			Rye flours (sifted):		
			Dark (1 cup)	4½ oz.	420
			Light (1 cup)	3¹⁄₁₀ oz.	315
			Medium (1 cup)	3¹⁄₁₀ oz.	310
			Soybean curd (tofu) (2½ × 2¾ × 1″)	4¼ oz.	85

° Calories listed for reference only. In practice, Calories are not counted for values less than 5.

ENERGY INTAKE TABLE, Continued

	Typical Measure	Calories (Rounded)		Typical Measure	Calories (Rounded)
Miscellaneous (Cooking Measures, Flour, Pastas, etc.), Cont.			**Nuts and Dried Seeds**		
			Almonds, roasted (10)	$\frac{9}{10}$ oz.	60
			Beans, dried:		
Soybean flours (stirred):			Black and brown		
Defatted (1 cup)	3½ oz.	325	(½ cup)	3¼ oz.	310
Full fat (1 cup)	2½ oz.	295	Calico (½ cup)	3¼ oz.	320
Low fat (1 cup)	3¹⁄₁₀ oz.	315	Kidney (½ cup)	3½ oz.	340
Spaghetti:			Lima (½ cup)	3½ oz.	340
Cooked, firm stage			Navy (½ cup)	3½ oz.	340
(1 cup)	4⅗ oz.	195	Pinto (½ cup)	3¼ oz.	320
Cooked, tender stage			Red (½ cup)	3½ oz.	340
(1 cup)	5 oz.	155	Red Mexican (½ cup)	3¼ oz.	320
With meatballs and			White (½ cup)	3½ oz.	340
tomato sauce (1 cup)	8¾ oz.	335	Brazil nuts, shelled (3)	1 oz.	90
With tomato sauce			Butternuts, shelled (9)	per oz.	180
and cheese (1 cup)	9 oz.	190	Cashew nuts, roasted		
Tapioca, dry (1 cup)	5⅓ oz.	535	(14 large, or 26 small)	per oz.	160
Tapioca, dry	1 T.	80	Chestnuts, in shell (10)	3 oz.	140
Tomato catsup	1 T.	15	Chestnuts, roasted		
Tomato chili sauce	1 T.	15	(1 cup)	5½ oz.	310
Tomato paste (1 cup)	9¼ oz.	215	Chick peas (¼ cup)	1¾ oz.	180
Welsh rarebit (1 cup)	8⅕ oz.	415	Coconut (1: 4⅝″ diam.)	27 oz.	1375
Wheat flour:			Meat, sliced		
All-purpose (1 cup)	4 oz.	420	(2 × 2 × ½″)	1½ oz.	155
Bread (1 cup)	4 oz.	420	Meat, grated or		
Cake or pastry (1 cup)	3⅓ oz.	350	shredded (1 cup,		
Gluten (1 cup: 45%			packed)	4½ oz.	450
gluten, 55% patent)	4¾ oz.	510	Milk (1 cup)	8½ oz.	605
Whole wheat (1 cup)	4 oz.	400	Cream	1 T.	50
Wheat germ	1 T.	23	Water (1 cup)	8½ oz.	55
Yeast:			Cow peas, dry (½ cup)	3 oz.	290
Baker's, compressed			Filberts (hazelnuts),		
(1 pkg.)	⅗ oz.	15	shelled (10)	1 oz.	85
Baker's, dry, active			Chopped	1 T.	45
(1 pkg. or T.)	¼ oz.	20	Garbanzo beans (¼ cup)	1¾ oz.	180
Brewer's, debittered			Hickory nuts, shelled		
(1 T.)	¼ oz.	23	(15)	½ oz.	100

	Typical Measure	Calories (Rounded)		Typical Measure	Calories (Rounded)
Lentils, dry (½ cup)	3⅖ oz.	325	Salads, cont.		
Litchi nuts, dried,			Fruit salad, canned,		
shelled (10)	5(+) oz.	70	water pack (½ cup)	4⅓ oz.	45
Macadamia nuts, shelled			Syrup pack (½ cup)	4½ oz.	100
(6)	½ oz.	110	Gelatin with fruit,		
Mixed nuts, shelled			no dressing (4″ sq.)	2 oz.	150
(8 to 10)	½ oz.	100	Potato salad (½ cup)	4⅖ oz.	150
Peanuts, chopped	1 T.	55	Seafood salad (1 cup)	6 oz.	400
Peanuts, roasted			Tomato aspic, mayon-		
(20 halves)	⅗ oz.	100	naise dressing (1 cup)	4 oz.	200
Pecans, shelled			Tuna salad (½ cup)	4 oz.	200
(12 halves)	½ oz.	100	Waldorf salad (½ cup)	2 oz.	150
Pine nuts, pignolias,			Salad ingredients:		
shelled	1 T.	45	Anchovies, pickled (5)	⅔ oz.	35
Pine nuts, pinon, shelled	1 T.	50	Anchovies, pickled	1 fillet	7
Pistachios, chopped	1 T.	55	Artichoke hearts	each	5
Pistachios, shelled (35)	⅗ oz.	100	Avocado (½ of 3⅛″ diam.)	4½ oz.	190
Pumpkin seeds, hulled			Bacon, crisp, whole		
(½ cup)	2½ oz.	385	or crumbled	½ oz.	50
Sesame seeds, hulled	1 T.	55	Banana, small		
Soybean seeds, dried			(7¾″ long), sliced	5 oz.	90
(½ cup)	3¾ oz.	425	Beets, pickled		
Walnuts, English,			(2″ diam.), sliced	2 oz.	15
shelled (10 halves)	½ oz.	100	Carrots, raw (½ cup)	2 oz.	25
			Cauliflower, raw (½ cup)	2 oz.	15
			Celery, raw, diced (½ cup)	2 oz.	10
Salads and Salad Ingredients			Chives, fresh chopped	1 T.	1
Salads			Cottage cheese	½ cup	125
(dressing included):			Cress, garden,		
Carrots and raisins			chopped	½ cup	12
(½ cup)	2 oz.	150	Cucumbers (8 slices:		
Chef's salad (1 cup)	4 oz.	400	⅛″ thick)	1 oz.	5
Chicken salad (½ cup)	4 oz.	200	Egg, medium,		
Cole slaw (1 cup)	3 oz.	100	hard-boiled	1	75
Crab Louis (1 cup)	6 oz.	400	Endive, escarole		
Dinner salad, side dish			(1 cup or 20 leaves)	2 oz.	10
(lettuce, tomato,			Fennel leaves		
dressing; 1 cup)	2 oz.	200	(1 cup)	2 oz.	10

ENERGY INTAKE TABLE, Continued

	Typical Measure	Calories (Rounded)		Typical Measure	Calories (Rounded)
Salads and Salad Ingredients, Cont.			Salad ingredients, cont.:		
Salad ingredients, cont.:			Chowchow, sweet		
Garlic	1 clove	5	(¼ cup)	2 oz.	70
Lemon juice	1 T.	3	Dill, whole		
Lettuce:			4″ long, 1¾″ diam.)	4¾ oz.	15
Butterhead (5″ head)	7¾ oz.	25	Dill, slices		
Crisphead (6″ head)	20 oz.	70	(2: 1½″ diam.)	¼ oz.	1
Looseleaf (1 cup)	2 oz.	10	Relish, sweet (1 T.)	½ oz.	20
Romaine or Cos			Sour, whole		
(1 cup)	2 oz.	10	(4″ long, 1¾″ diam.)	4¾ oz.	15
Macaroni, cold (½ cup)	2 oz.	100	Sour, slices		
Mushrooms (½ cup)	1 oz.	15	(2: 1½″ diam.)	¼ oz.	1
Olives (*quantity: size*):			Sweet, whole		
Green			(3″ long, 1″ diam.)	1¼ oz.	50
Giant			Small		
(*10*: ⅞″ diam.)	2¾ oz.	75	(2½″ long, ¾″ diam.)	½ oz.	25
Large			Radishes (*10*:		
(*10*: ⅚″ diam.)	1⅗ oz.	45	1″ diam.)	3 oz.	15
Small			Raisins (1 T.)	⅓ oz.	25
(*10*: ⅝″ diam.)	1⅖ oz.	35	Spinach (1 cup)	8⅖ oz.	45
Ripe:			Tomatoes, large:		
Ascalano, giant			(*1*: 3″ diam.)	7 oz.	40
(*10*: ¹³⁄₁₆″ diam.)	2⅘ oz.	90	Small (*1*: 2″ diam.)	4 oz.	25
Manzanilla, large			Salad dressings:		
(*10*: ¹⁵⁄₁₆″ diam.)	1⅔ oz.	50	Blue cheese	1 T.	80
Manzanilla, small			Caesar	1 T.	75
(*10*: ⅝″ diam.)	1⅖ oz.	40	French	1 T.	65
Mission, large			Garlic, creamy	1 T.	80
(*10*: ¾″ diam.)	1⅔ oz.	75	Green goddess	1 T.	75
Servillano,			Italian	1 T.	85
supercolossal			Lemon juice	1 T.	3
(*10*: 1¹⁄₁₆″ diam.)	5 oz.	115	Mayonnaise	1 T.	100
Pickles:			Olive oil	1 T.	125
Bread and butter			Roquefort	1 T.	80
slices (2: 1½″ diam.)	½ oz.	11	Russian	1 T.	75
Chowchow, sour			Thousand Island	1 T.	100
(¼ cup)	2 oz.	20	Vinegar	1 T.	2

	Typical Measure	Calories (Rounded)		Typical Measure	Calories (Rounded)
Sandwiches°			Chili	1 T.	20
Bacon and egg		400	Clam	1 T.	30
Bacon, lettuce and			Cranberry	1 T.	25
tomato		325	Gravy, beef	1 fl. oz.	25
Beef, barbecued		350	Gravy, chicken	1 fl. oz.	25
Beef, roast		300	Hollandaise	1 T.	100
Bologna		300	Horseradish	1 T.	10
Cheese		300	Lemon	1/4 cup	135
Cheeseburger		400	Lemon juice	1 oz.	6.5
Chicken, sliced or salad		300	Marinara	1 T.	20
Club, junior			Raisin	1/4 cup	125
(double deck)		350	Remoulade	1 T.	90
Club (triple deck)		450	Sour cream	1/4 cup	140
Corned beef		300	Soy	1 T.	10
Egg salad		300	Spaghetti meat sauce	1 T.	15
Ham and cheese		450	Spanish	1/2 cup	90
Ham, baked		400	Tartar	1 T.	100
Ham, boiled		350	Tomato	1 T.	20
Ham salad		300	Vinaigrette	1 T.	110
Hamburger		300	White sauce, thin	1 T.	20
Hotdog		300	Worcestershire	1 T.	10
Liverwurst		300			
Peanut butter (2 T.)		350	**Soups**		
Roast beef		300	Asparagus, cream of:		
Salami		300	Prepared with equal		
Tuna salad		300	parts of milk	1 cup	150
Turkey		300	Prepared with equal		
			parts of water	1 cup	65
Sauces and Gravies			Bean with bacon	1 cup	145
			Bean with pork	1 cup	170
Barbecue	1 T.	25	Beef	1 cup	90
Bearnaise	1 T.	60	Beef broth	1 cup	65
Bordelaise	1 T.	20	Beef noodle	1 cup	140
Catsup	1 T.	20	**Beef, vegetable with**		
Cheese	1 T.	35	barley	1 cup	65
			Black bean	1 cup	90
° Ingredients, in modest proportions, include			Borscht	1 cup	80
lettuce, tomato slice, pickle slices and dressings			Bouillon	1 cup	30
(1 T.).					

ENERGY INTAKE TABLE, Continued

	Typical Measure	Calories (Rounded)		Typical Measure	Calories (Rounded)
Soups, Cont.			Mushroom, cream of, cont.:		
Celery, cream of:			parts of milk	1 cup	215
Prepared with equal			Prepared with equal		
parts of milk	1 cup	175	parts of water	1 cup	135
Prepared with equal			Onion, cream of	1 cup	135
parts of water	1 cup	85	Onion, French	1 cup	65
Chicken, cream of:			Oxtail	1 cup	100
Prepared with equal			Oyster stew	1 cup	200
parts of milk	1 cup	180	Pea, green:		
Prepared with equal			Prepared with equal		
parts of water	1 cup	95	parts of milk	1 cup	215
Chicken gumbo	1 cup	115	Prepared with equal		
Chicken noodle	1 cup	130	parts of water	1 cup	130
Prepared with equal			Pea, split	1 cup	300
parts of water	1 cup	65	Prepared with equal		
Chicken vegetable	1 cup	155	parts of water	1 cup	145
Prepared with equal			Pepper pot	1 cup	85
parts of water	1 cup	75	Potato, cream of	1 cup	160
Chicken with rice	1 cup	95	Scotch broth	1 cup	75
Prepared with equal			Shrimp, cream of	1 cup	240
parts of water	1 cup	50	Tomato	1 cup	90
Clam chowder, Boston			Tomato, cream of	1 cup	175
(milk)	1 cup	160	Tomato, vegetable	1 cup	65
Clam chowder,			Tomato with rice	1 cup	95
Manhattan (tomato)	1 cup	60	Turkey, noodle	1 cup	160
Consomme, beef (with			Prepared with equal		
equal parts of water)	1 cup	30	parts of water	1 cup	80
Consomme, chicken (with			Turtle	1 cup	45
equal parts of water)	1 cup	20	Vegetable	1 cup	160
Gazpacho	1 cup	80	Prepared with equal		
Gumbo, creole	1 cup	60	parts of water	1 cup	80
Minestrone	1 cup	220	Vegetable beef	1 cup	165
Prepared with equal			Prepared with equal		
parts of water	1 cup	105	parts of water	1 cup	85
Mushroom, cream of:			Vichyssoise	1 cup	275
Prepared with equal			Won ton	1 cup	110

	Typical Measure	Calories (Rounded)		Typical Measure	Calories (Rounded)
Sugars and Sweets			**Vegetables**		
Jellies, jams and preserves:			Artichoke (edible portion: heart, under leaves)	1 bud (13½ oz.)	65
Apple butter	1 T.	35			
Chutney	1 T.	50	Artichoke hearts, canned	5	25
Guava butter	1 T.	40	Asparagus, large	each spear	5
Jams, assorted	1 T.	55			
Jellies, assorted	1 T.	50	Avocados (3⅛″ diam.)	½	185
Marmalade	1 T.	55	Bamboo shoots	1 cup	40
Peanut butter	1 T.	95	Bean sprouts, Mung	½ cup	15
Preserves, assorted	1 T.	50	Bean sprouts, Soy	½ cup	25
Sugar:			Beans:		
Brown, crude	1 T.	15	Baked with pork and sweet sauce	½ cup	190
Brown, dark	1 T.	50			
Maple	1 lump	50	Dried (*see* Nuts and Dried Seeds)		
Powdered	1 t., rounded	23	Green	½ cup	20
Powdered	1 T.	42	Kidney	½ cup	115
White, granular	1 t., level	15	Lima	½ cup	90
White, granular	1 t., rounded	32	Navy	½ cup	115
			Snap, green	½ cup	20
White, lump	1 piece	24	Soy	½ cup	40
Syrups:			String	½ cup	20
Apricot	1 T.	45	Wax	½ cup	20
Blackberry	1 T.	45	White	½ cup	115
Cane	1 T.	60	Yellow	½ cup	20
Chocolate	1 T.	50	Beets (2″ diam.), whole	2	30
Corn	1 T.	60	Sliced or diced	½ cup	30
Dextrose powder	1 T.	45	Blackeye peas	½ cup	90
Guava	1 T.	45	Broccoli:		
Honey	1 T.	65	Chopped	½ cup	25
Maple	1 T.	50	Large stalk	1	75
Molasses	1 T.	50	Small stalk	1	35
Papaya	1 T.	45	Brussels sprouts	4 sprouts (½ cup)	30
Raspberry	1 T.	45			
Strawberry	1 T.	45			

ENERGY INTAKE TABLE, Continued

	Typical Measure	Calories (Rounded)		Typical Measure	Calories (Rounded)
Vegetables, Cont.			Lentils, dried, cooked	½ cup	100
			Lettuce:		
Cabbage	1 cup	25	Butterhead		
Carrots			(e.g., Boston, Bibb)	5″ head	25
Raw (1″ diam.,			Crisphead (e.g., Ice-		
7″ long, 2½ oz.)	1	25	berg, N.Y. Great Lakes)	6″ head	10
Slices, raw or cooked	½ cup	25	Looseleaf (e.g., Grand		
Cauliflower	½ cup	15	Rapids, Salad Bowl,	1 cup	
Celery (4 oz. =			Simpson)	(2 oz.)	10
4 av. stalks = 1 cup)	1 cup	20	Romaine or Cos,	1 cup	
Chard, leaves	½ cup	15	chopped or shredded	(2 oz.)	10
Chervil	1 oz.	15	Mushrooms	½ cup	15
Chickpeas (garbanzos)	½ cup	360	Mustard greens	1 cup	30
Chives, chopped	1 T.	1	Mustard spinach	1 cup	30
Collards	½ cup	25	Okra	½ cup	30
Corn, canned	½ cup	100	Onions:		
Corn, fresh (ear:			Mature, chopped	1 T.	5
1¾″ diam., 5″ long)	1	70	Mature, chopped or		
Corn fritters			sliced	½ cup	30
(2″ diam., 1½″ thick)	1	130	Mature, whole		
Corn grits, cooked	½ cup	65	(2½″ diam.)	1	40
Cowpeas	½ cup	90	Young, green,		
Cucumbers	8 slices		chopped	½ cup	25
(⅛″ thick slices)	(1 oz.)	5	Young, green, whole		
Dandelion greens	1 cup	35	(small)	6	15
Eggplant	½ cup	20	Parsley, chopped		
Parmigiana			(10 sprigs, 2½″ long)	2 T.	5
(½″ thick slice)	1 fillet	200	Parsnips	½ cup	65
Scalloped			Peas	½ cup	65
(½″ thick slice)	1 fillet	100	Peas, mature, dried	½ cup	350
Endive	½ cup	5	Peppers:		
Escarole	½ cup	5	Hot, chili	2 T.	15
Garbanzos	½ cup	360	Mature, red (3″ diam. =		
Garlic	1 clove	5	1 cup sliced)	1	50
Grits, cooked	½ cup	65	Sweet, green (3″ diam.		
Hominy grits, cooked	½ cup	65	whole = 1 cup sliced)	1	35
Kale, leaves	½ cup	20	Pokeberry shoots	1 cup	35
Kohlrabi, diced	½ cup	20	Potato chips	each	10
Leeks	4	25	Potato salad	½ cup	150

	Typical Measure	Calories (Rounded)		Typical Measure	Calories (Rounded)
Potato sticks	1 cup	190	Rhubarb, diced, sugared	½ cup	195
Potatoes:			Rhubarb, diced,		
Au gratin	½ cup	175	unsweetened	½ cup	10
Baked (2 × 4″)	1	145	Rutabagas	½ cup	40
Boiled (2 × 4″)	1	175	Sauerkraut	½ cup	20
French fried			Spinach	1 cup	45
(3 to 4″ long)	each	20	Squash, summer	1 cup	30
Fried	½ cup	230	Squash, winter	1 cup	100
Hashed brown	½ cup	175	Tomatoes:		
Mashed (milk and			Canned	1 cup	50
table fat added)	½ cup	100	Large (3″ diam.; 7 oz.)	1	40
Scalloped,			Small (2″ diam.; 4 oz.)	1	25
with cheese	½ cup	175	Turnip greens	1 cup	30
Scalloped,			Turnips, cubed or sliced	1 cup	35
without cheese	½ cup	125	Turnips, mashed	1 cup	50
Potatoes, sweet:			Vegetables, mixed		
Baked (2 × 5″)	1	155	(succotash)	1 cup	115
Candied (2 × 2½″)	1	175	Water chestnuts	5 to 7	
Canned, mashed	½ cup	140	(1½″ diam., 4 oz.)	corms	70
Radishes (large:			Watercress	7 sprigs	5
1″ or more in diam.)	10	15			

Weights and Measures

The following tables present the weights and measures commonly used with foods in traditional U.S. units and in the International System of Units (Metric) adopted by the U.S. National Bureau of Standards in 1964. The relationships between the two systems are presented in practical equivalents. Volume and weight relationships depend on the substance (e.g., liquid or dry) measured. The weight and volume relationships presented for water help to establish a point of reference for comparing lighter (e.g., salad oils) or heavier liquids (e.g., syrups). Some household measuring units (e.g., the cup) commonly used with foods have not been officially recognized or adopted by the Bureau of Standards. Abbreviations are shown in parentheses. Each of the tables is organized from smaller (top) to larger (bottom) units and defined in terms of one unit of each measurement.

TABLE 11 **Weight**

Traditional U.S. Unit (Avoirdupois)	U.S. Equivalents	Metric Equivalents
grain	(0.036 drams)	64.799 milligrams (mg.)
dram	27.344 grains	1.722 grams (gm.)
ounce (oz.)	16 drams	28.350 gm.
pound (lb.)	16 oz.	453.592 gm.
		.454 kilograms (kg.)

Metric Unit	Metric Equivalents	Traditional U.S. Units
milligram (mg.)	1000 micrograms (mcg.)	
gram (gm.)	1000 mg.	.035 oz.
kilogram (kg.)	1000 gm.	2.2 lbs.

TABLE 12 **Volume, Liquid**

Traditional U.S. Unit	U.S. Equivalents	Metric Equivalents
teaspoon (t.)	(⅙ fl. oz.)	4.9 milliliters (ml.)
tablespoon (T.)	3 t.	14.8 ml.
fluid ounce (fl. oz.)	2 T.	29.573 ml.
cup (c.)	8 fl. oz.	237 ml.
pint (pt.)	2 cups	473 ml.; .473 liter
quart (qt.)	2 pints	.946 liter
gallon	4 quarts	3.785 liters

Metric Unit	Metric Equivalents	Traditional U.S. Units
liter (l.)	1000 milliliters (ml.)	1.06 quarts

TABLE 13 **Weight per Volume of Water**

Traditional U.S. Unit	U.S. Weight Equivalent	Metric Weight Equivalent
cubic centimeter (cc.)	.035 oz.	1 gm.
cup	8 oz.	237 gm.
quart	2 lb.	946 gm.

Metric Unit	Metric Weight Equivalent	U.S. Weight Equivalent
milliliter (ml.)	1 gm.	.035 oz.
liter (l.)	1 kg.	2.2 lb.

TABLE 14 **Conversion Factors for Weights and Measures**

To Change	to	Multiply by
Inches	Centimeters	2.54
Fluid ounces	Cubic centimeters	29.57
Quarts	Liters	.946
Cubic centimeters	Fluid ounces	.034
Liters	Quarts	1.057
Grains	Milligrams	64.799
Ounces (av.)	Grams	28.35
Pounds (av.)	Kilograms	.454
Kilograms	Pounds	2.205
Kilocalories	Kilojoules	4.181
Kilocalories	Megajoules	.004

Tips and Suggestions for Dieters

Reducing Rates

The higher the daily negative energy balance the faster the weight loss will be—up to a point. With a negative balance of 500 Calories you should lose about 1 pound of fat per week, or 3 to 4 pounds per month. A negative balance of 1000 should result in a loss of 6 to 8 pounds a month. Be prepared to lose more (fat weight plus fluid weight) at the beginning and less later, especially if you are also gaining lean tissue and muscle weight simultaneously through your fitness program. Don't be alarmed by day-to-day fluctuations, up or down; it is the long-term trend that is significant. There are many risks and discomforts connected with more severe reductions in food intake. A more rapid rate of weight loss is not recommended, and is less likely to be sustained than a gradual one involving behavior modification.

All Energy Values for Food and Physical Activity Are Approximate

Exact food values are affected by many factors and activity values depend greatly on the physical effort expended. The best way to use energy values effectively for purposes of weight control is to:

1. Use rounded numbers.
2. Understate energy output.
3. Overstate energy intake.
4. Consistently maintain negative energy balances.

Intake vs. Output

Many will argue that exercise is not necessary (it isn't) and that a reduction in diet is all that is needed (true). Nevertheless, even a modest exercise program (walking 30 minutes a day) will: (1) ease and speed a diet program by increasing metabolism; (2) help offset the loss of lean tissue that usually accompanies the loss of fat tissue during a diet; (3) promote good health and well being; and (4) keep body tissue firmer and appearance more attractive as fat decreases. If you think exercise makes you eat more, test your hypothesis. Most people eat less or even skip a meal following a vigorous exercise session.

Advertise Your Diet

Though you should not become a diet bore, it can aid your program to advertise it among your family, friends and associates. By reminding them that you need all the help you can get, you may at least discourage them from flaunting their own excessive indulgences. When dining out, you may fit in with the rest of the world by quietly eating smaller portions and avoiding extras, sauces and fats.

Avoid Temptations

Tempting foods, tempting places, appetizers (liquid or otherwise) and appetite stimulants of any kind should be avoided. People with a weight problem usually enjoy food more than others do and are stimulated by the sight, smell and availability of it. Try to keep food out of sight, out of mind—and inconvenient to obtain. Learn to anticipate, circumvent and defeat threats to your diet program: an empty stomach, periods of the day when your resistance is low, shopping or ordering food when hungry. Plan low-Calorie snacks or no-Calorie liquid fillers for between-meals periods or spread your daily intake over six small meals instead of three. Skip cocktail parties entirely or arrive at the last minute. But if a party is unavoidable, practice the dieter's dictum: Never eat or drink standing up—and don't sit down! If you need a glass to hold, use one filled with soda or mineral water. Then reward yourself with a tasty, low-Calorie prize after it's over. Most important of all: *Never let hunger sneak up on you and deprive you of self-control.* A slight, light snack prior to special events and dinner parties can be powerful preventive medicine.

Travel and Entertainment

The curse of the contemporary professional and business executive is expense-account living and the concomitant causes for eating and drinking too much: to celebrate a good day, to bury a bad one, to foster good fellowship, to lighten the burden of loneliness. It helps to develop specific strategies to cope with these situations, personal diet policies that you never allow yourself to violate. On the road and eating out are good times to brush up on Calorie counting, double-checking memorized counts, adding new ones. Coping tactics include mineral waters instead of cocktails, soups or salads or sea-food cocktails instead of entrees, adding up your energy intake for the day *before* dinner and limiting yourself to the balance, ordering foods you don't particularly like, talking more than eating or drinking (using your hands to gesture a lot).

Profit from Mistakes

Binges and breakdowns in your diet should be viewed as mistakes and temporary setbacks. Use them to improve your knowledge of yourself and the way your diet works for you. Why did you break your diet? Did you allow hunger to sway judgment? Were you overpowered by fatigue or environmental stimulation? Has your diet become too repetitive and monotonous? Use the mistakes to learn new behavior patterns that will help you to control your diet and prevent them in the future.

Be Prepared for Plateaus

As fat is lost, water accumulates. If you are exercising regularly you may be replacing fat weight with heavier muscle, bone and blood weight. If you have lost more than 2 pounds a week you tend to gain back the extra pounds before resuming the downward trend.

Eat Smaller Bites More Slowly and Enjoy Each of Them More

Soon you may discover that *less is more* as you savor each bite with distinct pleasure and relish. Give your body a chance to send and receive signals of satiation. When you eat in a hurry the food can already be in your stomach and the damage done by the time you get the message that you are no longer hungry. Food tastes much better in your mouth—and not at all in your stomach. For the same reasons, never eat standing up.

Keep Records of What and How Much You Eat

Calories *do* count whether the people who use energy count them or not. But there may be reason to believe that *differences in body mechanisms* and the *nutrient mix in the diet itself* can make a difference in the rates at which a person uses, loses and keeps energy. Experiments have shown that variations in the proportions of proteins, fats and carbohydrates contained in diets having the same total energy content can make a difference in weight maintenance.[*] Therefore, if your energy log records a substantial daily negative balance over a long period of time (a month or more) but no corresponding loss in body weight, you should discuss the content of your diet with your adviser. If may be that a different nutrient mix will improve your results.

Fasting and Starvation Are Not Recommended

The body uses carbohydrates for energy in preference to both fat and protein, but the amount of carbohydrates stored in the body (mostly in the liver and the muscles) is limited to less than one day's supply. After the first few hours of starvation, during which time the carbohydrate supply is exhausted, the body starts burning *both* tissue fat and protein. Losing the fat is fine. Losing the protein is not so good. To avoid these problems and to be on the safe side, physiologists recommend *daily* intake of 50 grams to as much as 75 grams of protein, or one gram of protein per kilogram of body weight.

Even if starvation and fasting were not proven by experimental tests to be harmful, there are additional experimental results which indicate that fasting is actually *counter-productive* to long-term weight control and fat reduction. The reasons for this, apparently, lie in the amazing defense systems and strategies of the body. The body adapts to long-term food deprivation by increasing fat deposits so that the next time fasting is at-

[*] See D. S. Miller and P. R. Payne: "Weight Maintenance and Food Intake." *Journal of Nutrition*, 78: 225 (1962); D. S. Miller and P. Munford: "Gluttony. An Experimental Study of Overeating in Low- or High-Protein Diets." *American Journal of Clinical Nutrition*, 20: 1212 (1967); R. Schemmel, "Food Product Development," July/August 1975; and other studies including those of L. M. Zucker (1975) and C. M. Young, S. S. Scanlan and H. Im (1971).

tempted the body can—and does—retain fat longer than it did the first time.°

In the final analysis gimmicks, quick cures and extreme dietary solutions are both deceptive and dangerous. Spectacular battles may be won or lost daily, but the war against excess fat is ultimately and permanently won by a long, steady, methodical change in energy use habits and control.

Low-Carbohydrate Diets

When excessive carbohydrates are taken in, fats can be synthesized instead of being degraded, thereby *increasing* instead of *reducing* the stored fat. Therefore, a low-carbohydrate diet is widely believed to be especially desirable. However, too low a level of carbohydrate intake can cause trouble. Adequate carbohydrates are necessary for proper functioning of the kidneys and to avoid acidosis (too much acid in the blood).

Carbohydrates are the starchy foods and sugars that may be reduced to lower intake levels most easily by:

1. Avoiding desserts with meals and sweet snacks between meals.
2. Eliminating sugar in drinks.

A daily intake of 70 to 100 grams of carbohydrates is sufficient to meet your nutritional needs. Each of the following would provide the entire allotment of grams for the day:

Five 6-oz. bottles of carbonated drinks
Four glasses of cider or lemonade
Four pieces of whole fruit (apple, peach, pear)
Two large (3-oz.) candy bars
Two slices (4″ wedge) of pie
One generous (3″ wedge) slice of cake with icing
One cup of macaroni

° See J. Mayer *et al.*: "Symposium: Feeding Patterns and Their Biochemical Consequences." *Fed. Proc.* 23: 59 (1964); and P. Fabry: "Metabolic Consequences of the Pattern of Food Intake" in D. F. Code: *Handbook of Physiology*, Williams and Wilkins, 1967.

From a practical standpoint, you may obtain all the carbohydrates you need from the cereals, vegetables, milk and bread that should be a part of your normal diet. The foods to avoid are sugar, syrups, molasses, honey, candy, cake, cookies, cream, puddings, pies, sugar-sweetened drinks and alcoholic beverages.

Cholesterol and Triglycerides

An excess of fatty substances (lipids called *cholesterol* and *triglycerides*) in the blood is believed to be a major contributor to coronary artery disease. To control intake of these elements in your diet to one-third of the total, as you should for good nutrition, eat:

- Polyunsaturated margarine and vegetable oils instead of saturated fats
- Lean cuts of meat (trim all visible fat)
- Fish
- No-fat or low-fat dairy products

Eat less:

- Sugars, syrups, jellies, honey
- Candy, cookies and cakes

And, as much as possible, eat no:

- Egg yolks (maximum: three per week)
- Animal organs
- Sausage meats
- Shrimp
- Whole milk dairy products
- Fatty cuts of meat

Vitamins and Minerals

Vitamins and minerals are essential to good health. The best way to assure adequate intake is to eat a wide variety of foods and a liberal supply of non-fat milk, meat, fruit and vegetables.

Hunger-Satisfying Foods

No matter what we call it, dieting to lose weight is partial starvation and rarely enjoyed by those who need it the most. It is important, therefore, to keep the dieter as comfortable as possible. Serving foods that satisfy helps to accomplish this purpose. Such foods should be included with each meal, if possible. Foods with high satiety value that seem to "stick to the ribs" include meat, poultry, fish and dairy products. Fats, which leave the stomach last, should also be included with each meal. Eating smaller portions more frequently helps greatly to mask the semi-starvation process. A teaspoon of polyunsaturated vegetable oil salad dressing can convert a half-head of lettuce into a glutton's delight at an energy intake cost of less than 100 Calories. A *small* fish or poultry entree surrounded by a plate loaded with green beans and carrots can be interesting and filling at a cost of no more than 300 Calories. Raw celery and carrots in heaping quantities can be as pleasing as a bowl full of salted nuts at a fraction of the Calorie count. Fruit can be used to replace fattening desserts and in-between meal snacks. Herbs and spices can dress up foods without increasing the intake cost at all.

Record Keeping

Keep your diary going no matter what happens to your performance. The continuation of your diary is a powerful stimulant to successful behavior modification. An honest, accurate record of your uses of energy can help you identify and correct mistakes.

PART II

The Fitness and Weight Control Program

Beginning with this section of the book, you start writing and I stop. These remaining pages are designed to assist you in establishing a systematic fitness and weight control program by enabling you to write, as promised on page 1, "your own prescription for diet and exercise, eating foods you like and doing activities you enjoy." What you write in these pages may be drawn, and adapted, from the information provided in the first part of the book.

The next few pages provide *summary forms* for your convenience. These forms will help you summarize the information in the first part of the book that you will use the most, and most frequently, in keeping your diary.

1. *Fitness and Weight Control Profile* (page 79). This form summarizes your own personal measurements and goals. By now, you probably have already written the information you need in the blanks provided.

2. *Energy Output Summary* (page 82). You may use this form to transfer those activities in which you *normally* engage on a day-to-day basis. Once it is completed, you will need to consult the Energy Output Table in the first section (pages 15–19) only when you are undertaking an unusual activity not listed in your Summary.

3. *Energy Intake Summary* (page 83). This quick calorie counter presents on one page a complete guide to all foods that may be used for reliable estimates of energy values.

4. *Daily Energy Control Summary* (page 84). This worksheet summarizes the recommendations of most nutritionists and provides space to plan your own dietary allowances.

5. *Personal Diet Food List* (page 87). Using this form you may list your favorites in each food category for planning menus and for convenient reference when eating out. Once it is completed, the more extensive Energy Intake Table (pages 38–67) need be consulted only when you consider foods not included in your regular diet.

6. *Fitness and Weight Control Program Summary* (page 92). This form will enable you to summarize and review your progress using the essential weight, daily energy balance and fitness measurement results recorded in your diary. This form may be especially useful for periodic consultations with your doctor or dietician.

AFTERWORD

By the time you reach this page your program should be well under way. I hope you find this opportunity to study your own body and its uses of energy as interesting as I found studying mine when I was forced to reduce my weight. Your fitness and weight control program should be a grand opportunity to play scientist, learn more about yourself, and to reform your attitudes and habits for a happier, healthier, longer life. If your experience is like mine, you'll enjoy it—so why rush? Take your time. It's pleasanter to lose weight at a leisurely pace. Good luck.

FITNESS AND WEIGHT CONTROL PROFILE

Name _____

Sex _____ Height _____ Age _____

Present weight: _____

Skinfold measurements: Abdomen _____ Arm _____

       Back _____ Chest _____ Hip _____ Thigh _____

Body fat percentage _____

Ideal weight _____

Resting Metabolic Rate _____

Occupational group _____ Vigor level _____

Estimated Daily Energy Requirement _____

Maximum heart rate _____

Target zone for pulse-rated exercise _____ to _____

Fitness program goals and special considerations _____

_____

_____

_____

_____

Weight control goals and special considerations _____

_____

_____

_____

_____

_____

_____

Example 2

ENERGY OUTPUT SUMMARY

Energy Output	Calories (Rounded)	
Resting Metabolic Rate 1692		
Estimated Daily Energy Requirement 2200 ◀		— **Number of Calories Rounded**
Daily Activities:		
Sleep & TV in Bed	70 ◀	
Sit, Read, Watch TV	85	
Office Work	100	
Driving	100 ◀	
Standing & Moving	120	**Calorie Count**
Dressing	120 ◀	**Adjusted Downward**
House Work	130	
Eating	150	
Playing Piano	160	
Walking Slowly	200	
		Number of Activities Limited
Fitness Activities:		
Walking Briskly	245	
Cycling – 5 to 10 mph	280	
Cycling – 10 mph	415	

Energy Output Summary

It will be easier to keep track of your energy output if you summarize the activities in which you regularly engage, transferring the ones you checked in the Energy Output Table. Example 2 shows such a summary for a 50-year-old business executive. Note that:

1. The Calorie counts have been *rounded* to simplify calculations.
2. The number of activities has been *limited* to a practical amount.
3. The Calorie counts for *driving* and for *dressing* have been adapted and reduced to conform to lower expectations for energy usage.

Before completing your own summary on the next page, take a look at a daily log kept by our 50-year-old business executive (Example 3) to see how this information may be used.

EXAMPLE 3

Date: Wgt. Day 21

Hr.	Energy Output Log	Cal.
	Sleep 7 x 70	490
	Cycle ½ x 415	210
	Dress ¼ x 120	30
	Eat ¼ x 150	40
	Drive 1 x 100	100
	Office 3 x 100	300
	Lunch 1 x 150	150
	Office 5 x 100	500
	Drive 1 x 100	100
	Dinner	150
	Reading 3 x 85	255
	Sleep	70
		2395

Total Out

ENERGY OUTPUT SUMMARY

	Calories (Rounded)
Energy Output	
Resting Metabolic Rate	
Estimated Daily Energy Requirement	
Daily Activities:	
Fitness Activities:	

Note in Example 3 that:

1. Calorie counts are *rounded* for ease in calculations.
2. Activities are *summarized* and kept mostly on the basis of an hour or more.
3. More precise time measurement is kept for *fitness activity.*
4. This person exceeded his estimated Daily Energy Requirement by an output of 195 Calories (2395 vs. an estimated Daily Energy Requirement of 2200). All, or almost all, of the excess appears to be attributable to the fitness exercise on the bicycle. (If he restricts energy intake to 1395 Calories on a diet regimen he can lose two pounds a week at this rate.)

Energy Intake Summary

This quick Calorie counter presents a complete guide to all foods that may be used for reliable estimates of energy values when there isn't time

ENERGY INTAKE SUMMARY

Food	Calories (Rounded) Per Serving	Food	Calories (Rounded) Per Serving
Beverages:		Fruit and fruit juice	100
Alcoholic	150	Meat, fish and game	
Dairy	200	(3 to 5 oz.)	400
Non-alcoholic	100	Nuts and seeds	150
Breads	75	Salads:	
With butter or margarine	100	With dressing	350
Breakfast cereals, hot or cold:		Without dressing	100
with milk and sugar	300	Sandwiches	400
with milk, no sugar	250	Sauces, gravies or toppings	100
Cheese	100	Soup:	
Crackers	100	Thick (e.g., vegetable)	150
Desserts	400	Thin (e.g., broth)	75
Eggs (each)	100	Sugar syrups or sweets added	50
Fats and oils, animal or		Vegetables:	
vegetable	125	Leafy, green and yellow	25
		Starchy	100

for more detailed analysis, or by serious dieters who wish to conduct a weight control program using a minimum of numerical information. See the Energy Intake Table (pages 38–67) for more detailed Caloric values for specific foods. The portions described are assumed to be modest, diet-conscious portions.

Daily Energy Control Summary

The Daily Energy Control Summary is a worksheet that summarizes the recommendations of most nutritionists and dieticians and provides space to plan your own diet. The first two columns of the Summary indicate

DAILY ENERGY CONTROL SUMMARY

Food Categories	No. of Servings	Calories per Serving (Low)	Calories per Serving (High)	Col 1 × 2 (Low)	Col 1 × 3 (High)	Your Diet Program
			Recommendations for Low-Calorie Diets			
1. Appetizers and snacks		25	150			_____
2. Beverages		0	150			_____
3. Breads or cereals	3	50	75	150	225	_____
4. Milk, cheese or eggs	2	80	100	160	200	_____
5. Butter, margarine or oil	3	50	75	150	225	_____
6. Desserts & sweet snacks		50	150			_____
7. Fruit	2	50	100	100	200	_____
8. Meat, fish or game (3 oz.)	2	150	300	300	600	_____
9. Nuts and nibbles		50	100			_____
10. Salads, no dressing	2	25	50	50	100	_____
with dressing		2	50			_____
11. Soup	2	20	75	40	150	_____
12. Vegetables	2+	25	50	50	100	_____
Energy Intake Allowance				+1000	+1800	_____
Daily Energy Requirement				−2000	−2800	_____
Energy Balance				−1000	−1000	_____

DAILY ENERGY CONTROL SUMMARY, Continued

Line Notes for Dieters

1. Low-Calorie substitutes include carrots, cauliflower, celery, radishes, bouillon.
2. Use as desired: coffee and tea (without milk or sugar), lemon juice and mineral waters. Fruit and vegetable juices have low energy costs.
3. Stress whole grains. Eliminate jellies, syrup, sugar.
4. Use non-fat (skim) milk.
5. 1 t. butter, margarine or vegetable oil (less than 50 Cal. each) with vegetables or salads aids feeling of satiety. Use freely: herbs, vinegar, lemon juice.
6. Substitute fruits or diet portions if you cannot avoid entirely.
7. Fresh fruits and canned or stewed fruits without sugar.
8. Stress lean meats, fish, cottage cheese. Avoid fried and fatty meats. Trim all visible fat.
9. Substitute low- (and no) Calorie chews: raw carrots, cauliflower, celery, radishes.
10. Gourmand's salad (50 Cal.): One whole 7¾ oz., 5-inch head of Butterhead lettuce sprinkled with herbs, 1 t. polyunsaturated vegetable oil, lemon juice, tossed.
11. Stress clear soups. If too much soup, exchange freely for leafy, green and yellow vegetables.
12. No penalties for extra-large servings of watery and fibrous, leafy, green and yellow vegetables. Count corn, peas, dried beans under #3.
13. The Bottom Line: Average woman loses up to 2 pounds per week ($+1000 - 2000 = -1000 = -2$ pounds); average man loses up to 2 pounds per week ($+1800 - 2800 = -1000 = -2$ pounds).

nutritionists' recommendations for daily servings in each food category, some of which were presented earlier in Table 9. A blank means none is recommended. The next two columns indicate the number of Calories recommended per serving for low-Calorie diets, ranging from 1000 to 1800 Calories per day. Most weight reduction diets fall within a range of 1000 to 1500 Calories (including those that claim Calories don't count).

Use the last column of the Summary to write in your own daily diet allowance. Then add up your total Energy Intake Allowance and subtract your Daily Energy Requirement to see how many pounds a week you may lose on your personal diet regimen.

Personal Diet Food List

On the pages that follow, list your favorites in each food category of your diet and indicate the serving measure that fits the Calorie level of your personal diet. This will help you to select foods and plan meals you like more quickly and easily.

Example 4 on the next page shows a sample food list for a diet allowance of 1800 Calories daily.

EXAMPLE 4

PERSONAL DIET FOOD LIST

Food Category: Breads & Cereals   Food Category: _____

1 serving = 75 Calories ____   1 serving = _____ Calories ____

FOOD	SERVING MEASURE	FOOD	SERVING MEASURE
Bagel	½ Piece	Spaghetti	½ Cup
Boston Brown Bread	1 Slice		
English Muffin	½		
Flat Bread	3½ Wafers		
Bread	1 Slice		
Melba Toast	5 Slices		
Zweiback	2 Slices		
Cereals:			
40% Bran	⅔ Cup		
Corn Flakes	¾ Cup		
Puffed Rice	1 Cup		
Wheat Flakes	⅔ Cup		
Cream of Wheat	½ Cup		
Oatmeal	½ Cup		
Crackers:			
Rye (2"×3")	3		
Wheat (2" sq.)	3		

PERSONAL DIET FOOD LIST

Food Category: _____ | *Food Category:* _____
1 serving = _____ *Calories* ____ | *1 serving =* _____ *Calories* ____

FOOD	SERVING MEASURE	FOOD	SERVING MEASURE

PERSONAL DIET FOOD LIST, Continued

Food Category: _____
1 serving = _____ *Calories* ____

Food Category: _____
1 serving = _____ *Calories* ____

FOOD	SERVING MEASURE	FOOD	SERVING MEASURE

| Food Category: _____ | | Food Category: _____ | |
| 1 serving = _____ Calories ___ | | 1 serving = _____ Calories ___ | |
FOOD	SERVING MEASURE	FOOD	SERVING MEASURE

PERSONAL DIET FOOD LIST, Continued

Food Category: _____ 1 serving = _____ Calories ____		Food Category: _____ 1 serving = _____ Calories ____	
FOOD	SERVING MEASURE	FOOD	SERVING MEASURE

Food Category: _____ | *Food Category:* _____
1 serving = _____ *Calories* ____ | *1 serving =* _____ *Calories* ____

FOOD	SERVING MEASURE	FOOD	SERVING MEASURE

FITNESS AND WEIGHT CONTROL PROGRAM SUMMARY

Day	Weight	Energy Balance	Fitness Measurement
1			
2			
3			
4			
5			
6			
7			
8			
9			
10			
11			
12			
13			
14			
15			
16			
17			
18			
19			
20			
21			
22			
23			
24			
25			
26			

Day	Weight	Energy Balance	Fitness Measurement
27			
28			
29			
30			
31			
32			
33			
34			
35			
36			
37			
38			
39			
40			
41			
42			

Calories In
Calories Out

Date:	Wgt.	Day **1**		Date:	Wgt.	Day **2**	
Hr.	**Energy Output Log**		**Cal.**	**Hr.**	**Energy Output Log**		**Cal.**
		Total Out				**Total Out**	
	Energy Input Log		**Cal.**		**Energy Input Log**		**Cal.**
Break: ☐				Break: ☐			
Lunch: ☐				Lunch: ☐			
Dinner: ☐				Dinner: ☐			

Fitness Log

		Total In (+)				Total In (+)	
		Total Out (−)				Total Out (−)	
		Balance (±)				Balance (±)	

☑ = check when medication is taken.

Calories In
Calories Out

| Date: | Wgt. | Day | **3** | Date: | Wgt. | Day | **4** |

Hr.	Energy Output Log	Cal.	Hr.	Energy Output Log	Cal.
	Total Out			**Total Out**	
	Energy Input Log	Cal.		Energy Input Log	Cal.
	Break: ☐			Break: ☐	
	Lunch: ☐			Lunch: ☐	
	Dinner: ☐			Dinner: ☐	

Fitness Log

		Total In (+)			Total In (+)
		Total Out (−)			Total Out (−)
		Balance (±)			Balance (±)

☑ = check when medication is taken.

Calories In / Calories Out

				5					6

Date: _____ Wgt. _____ Day **5**   Date: _____ Wgt. _____ Day **6**

Hr.	Energy Output Log	Cal.	Hr.	Energy Output Log	Cal.
		Total Out			**Total Out**

Energy Input Log	Cal.	Energy Input Log	Cal.
Break: ☐		Break: ☐	
Lunch: ☐		Lunch: ☐	
Dinner: ☐		Dinner: ☐	

Fitness Log				Fitness Log			
		Total In (+)				Total In (+)	
		Total Out (−)				Total Out (−)	
		Balance (±)				Balance (±)	

☑ = check when medication is taken.

7

| | | | 8 |

Date: Wgt. Day **7**   Date: Wgt. Day **8**

Hr.	Energy Output Log	Cal.	Hr.	Energy Output Log	Cal.
	Total Out			**Total Out**	

Energy Input Log	Cal.	Energy Input Log	Cal.
Break: ☐		Break: ☐	
Lunch: ☐		Lunch: ☐	
Dinner: ☐		Dinner: ☐	

Fitness Log   Fitness Log

		Total In (+)			Total In (+)
		Total Out (−)			Total Out (−)
		Balance (±)			Balance (±)

☑ = check when medication is taken.

Calories In Calories Out

Date:	Wgt.	Day **9**		Date:	Wgt.	Day **10**

Hr.	Energy Output Log	Cal.	Hr.	Energy Output Log	Cal.
		Total Out			**Total Out**

Energy Input Log	Cal.	Energy Input Log	Cal.
Break: ☐		Break: ☐	
Lunch: ☐		Lunch: ☐	
Dinner: ☐		Dinner: ☐	
Fitness Log		Fitness Log	

		Total In (+)			Total In (+)
		Total Out (−)			Total Out (−)
		Balance (±)			Balance (±)

☑ = check when medication is taken.

Calories In
Calories Out

		11					12

Date: Wgt.   Day **11**   Date: Wgt.   Day **12**

Hr.	Energy Output Log	Cal.	Hr.	Energy Output Log	Cal.
	Total Out			**Total Out**	

Energy Input Log	Cal.	Energy Input Log	Cal.
Break: ☐		Break: ☐	
Lunch: ☐		Lunch: ☐	
Dinner: ☐		Dinner: ☐	

Fitness Log   Fitness Log

		Total In (+)				Total In (+)	
		Total Out (−)				Total Out (−)	
		Balance (±)				Balance (±)	

☑ = check when medication is taken.

Calories In Calories Out

| Date: | Wgt. | Day **13** | Date: | Wgt. | Day **14** |

Hr.	Energy Output Log	Cal.	Hr.	Energy Output Log	Cal.
	Total Out			**Total Out**	

	Energy Input Log	Cal.		Energy Input Log	Cal.
Break: ☐			Break: ☐		
Lunch: ☐			Lunch: ☐		
Dinner: ☐			Dinner: ☐		

Fitness Log

		Total In (+)			Total In (+)
		Total Out (−)			Total Out (−)
		Balance (±)			Balance (±)

☑ = check when medication is taken.

	15			16
Date: Wgt. Day **15**   Date: Wgt. Day **16**

Hr.	Energy Output Log	Cal.	Hr.	Energy Output Log	Cal.

Total Out

Energy Input Log	Cal.	Energy Input Log	Cal.
Break: ☐		Break: ☐	
Lunch: ☐		Lunch: ☐	
Dinner: ☐		Dinner: ☐	

Fitness Log

		Total In (+)			Total In (+)
		Total Out (−)			Total Out (−)
		Balance (±)			Balance (±)

☑ = check when medication is taken.

Calories In Calories Out

| Date: | Wgt. | Day **17** | Date: | Wgt. | Day **18** |

Hr.	Energy Output Log	Cal.	Hr.	Energy Output Log	Cal.

Total Out **Total Out**

Energy Input Log	Cal.	Energy Input Log	Cal.
Break: ☐		Break: ☐	
Lunch: ☐		Lunch: ☐	
Dinner: ☐		Dinner: ☐	

Fitness Log **Fitness Log**

		Total In (+)				Total In (+)	
		Total Out (−)				Total Out (−)	
		Balance (±)				Balance (±)	

☑ = check when medication is taken.

		19				**20**
Date:	Wgt.	Day	Date:	Wgt.	Day	

Hr.	Energy Output Log	Cal.	Hr.	Energy Output Log	Cal.
	Total Out			Total Out	
	Energy Input Log	Cal.		Energy Input Log	Cal.
Break: ☐			Break: ☐		
Lunch: ☐			Lunch: ☐		
Dinner: ☐			Dinner: ☐		
Fitness Log			Fitness Log		

		Total In (+)			Total In (+)
		Total Out (−)			Total Out (−)
		Balance (±)			Balance (±)

☑ = check when medication is taken.

21 **22**

| Date: | Wgt. | Day | | Date: | Wgt. | Day | |

Hr.	Energy Output Log	Cal.	Hr.	Energy Output Log	Cal.

Total Out **Total Out**

Energy Input Log	Cal.	Energy Input Log	Cal.
Break: ☐		Break: ☐	
Lunch: ☐		Lunch: ☐	
Dinner: ☐		Dinner: ☐	

Fitness Log **Fitness Log**

		Total In (+)				Total In (+)	
		Total Out (−)				Total Out (−)	
		Balance (±)				Balance (±)	

☑ = check when medication is taken.

Calories In
Calories Out

| Date: | Wgt. | Day | **23** | Date: | Wgt. | Day | **24** |

Hr.	Energy Output Log	Cal.		Hr.	Energy Output Log	Cal.

	Total Out				Total Out	
Energy Input Log		Cal.		Energy Input Log		Cal.
Break: ☐				Break: ☐		
Lunch: ☐				Lunch: ☐		
Dinner: ☐				Dinner: ☐		

Fitness Log				Fitness Log		
		Total In (+)				Total In (+)
		Total Out (−)				Total Out (−)
		Balance (±)				Balance (±)

☑ = check when medication is taken.

Date:	Wgt.	Day	**25**	Date:	Wgt.	Day	**26**

Hr.	Energy Output Log	Cal.	Hr.	Energy Output Log	Cal.

Total Out

Energy Input Log	Cal.	Energy Input Log	Cal.
Break: ☐		Break: ☐	
Lunch: ☐		Lunch: ☐	
Dinner: ☐		Dinner: ☐	

Fitness Log

		Total In (+)			Total In (+)
		Total Out (−)			Total Out (−)
		Balance (±)			Balance (±)

☑ = check when medication is taken.

			27				**28**
Date:	Wgt.	Day		Date:	Wgt.	Day	

Hr.	Energy Output Log	Cal.	Hr.	Energy Output Log	Cal.
		Total Out			**Total Out**	

Energy Input Log	Cal.	Energy Input Log	Cal.
Break: ☐		Break: ☐	
Lunch: ☐		Lunch: ☐	
Dinner: ☐		Dinner: ☐	

Fitness Log				Fitness Log			
		Total In (+)				Total In (+)	
		Total Out (−)				Total Out (−)	
		Balance (±)				Balance (±)	

☑ = check when medication is taken.

Date:	Wgt.	Day **29**		Date:	Wgt.	Day **30**	

Hr.	Energy Output Log	Cal.	Hr.	Energy Output Log	Cal.
	Total Out			**Total Out**	

Energy Input Log	Cal.	Energy Input Log	Cal.
Break: ☐		Break: ☐	
Lunch: ☐		Lunch: ☐	
Dinner: ☐		Dinner: ☐	
Fitness Log		**Fitness Log**	

		Total In (+)			Total In (+)
		Total Out (−)			Total Out (−)
		Balance (±)			Balance (±)

☑ = check when medication is taken.

| Date: | Wgt. | Day | **31** | Date: | Wgt. | Day | **32** |

Hr.	Energy Output Log	Cal.		Hr.	Energy Output Log	Cal.
	Total Out				**Total Out**	
	Energy Input Log	Cal.			Energy Input Log	Cal.
Break: ☐				Break: ☐		
Lunch: ☐				Lunch: ☐		
Dinner: ☐				Dinner: ☐		

Fitness Log			Fitness Log	
		Total In (+)			Total In (+)
		Total Out (−)			Total Out (−)
		Balance (±)			Balance (±)

☑ = check when medication is taken.

**Calories In
Calories Out**

| Date: | Wgt. | Day **33** | Date: | Wgt. | Day **34** |

Hr.	Energy Output Log	Cal.	Hr.	Energy Output Log	Cal.

	Total Out			Total Out	
Energy Input Log		Cal.	Energy Input Log		Cal.
Break: ☐			Break: ☐		
Lunch: ☐			Lunch: ☐		
Dinner: ☐			Dinner: ☐		
Fitness Log			Fitness Log		

		Total In (+)				Total In (+)	
		Total Out (−)				Total Out (−)	
		Balance (±)				Balance (±)	

☑ = check when medication is taken.

Date:	Wgt. Day **35**		Date:	Wgt. Day **36**	
Hr.	Energy Output Log	Cal.	Hr.	Energy Output Log	Cal.
	Total Out			**Total Out**	
	Energy Input Log	Cal.		Energy Input Log	Cal.
	Break: ☐			Break: ☐	
	Lunch: ☐			Lunch: ☐	
	Dinner: ☐			Dinner: ☐	

Fitness Log | | | | **Fitness Log** | |

		Total In (+)			Total In (+)
		Total Out (−)			Total Out (−)
		Balance (±)			Balance (±)

☑ = check when medication is taken.

Calories In Calories Out

| Date: | Wgt. | Day **37** | Date: | Wgt. | Day **38** |

Hr.	Energy Output Log	Cal.	Hr.	Energy Output Log	Cal.
	Total Out			**Total Out**	

Energy Input Log	Cal.	Energy Input Log	Cal.
Break: ☐		Break: ☐	
Lunch: ☐		Lunch: ☐	
Dinner: ☐		Dinner: ☐	

Fitness Log

		Total In (+)			Total In (+)
		Total Out (−)			Total Out (−)
		Balance (±)			Balance (±)

☑ = check when medication is taken.

| Date: | Wgt. | Day | **39** | Date: | Wgt. | Day | **40** |

Hr.	Energy Output Log	Cal.		Hr.	Energy Output Log	Cal.
	Total Out				**Total Out**	

Energy Input Log	Cal.		Energy Input Log	Cal.
Break: ☐			Break: ☐	
Lunch: ☐			Lunch: ☐	
Dinner: ☐			Dinner: ☐	

Fitness Log			Fitness Log		
		Total In (+)			Total In (+)
		Total Out (−)			Total Out (−)
		Balance (±)			Balance (±)

☑ = check when medication is taken.

Calories In
Calories Out

			41				**42**
Date:	Wgt.	Day		Date:	Wgt.	Day	

Hr.	Energy Output Log	Cal.	Hr.	Energy Output Log	Cal.
	Total Out			**Total Out**	
	Energy Input Log	Cal.		**Energy Input Log**	Cal.
Break: ☐			Break: ☐		
Lunch: ☐			Lunch: ☐		
Dinner: ☐			Dinner: ☐		
Fitness Log			**Fitness Log**		

		Total In (+)			Total In (+)
		Total Out (−)			Total Out (−)
		Balance (±)			Balance (±)

☑ = check when medication is taken.

INDEX

Be sure you also have

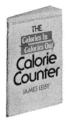

THE CALORIES IN/CALORIES OUT
CALORIE COUNTER
The Calorie Counter that Counts Both Ways
by James Leisy

In a handy, carry-along size, this book provides extensive lists of the calories-out counts for hundreds of activities from typing to housepainting, and the calories-in counts for hundreds of generic and name-brand foods and beverages. This is the watchdog that makes it possible to monitor diet and exercise all day, every day, everywhere—and to maintain the optimum in-out energy balance for lasting fitness.

The salient points of Leisy's program are covered, including the vital formulas for computing individual Resting Metabolic Rate and Daily Energy Requirement. Includes a two-week supply of diary pages.

Paperback, $3.95

from your favorite bookseller, or
directly from
THE STEPHEN GREENE PRESS
Brattleboro, VT 05301